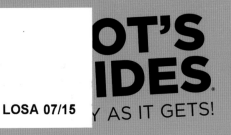

Nail Art

by Emily Draher

ALPHA

A member of Penguin Group (USA) Inc.

ALPHA BOOKS

Published by Penguin Group (USA) Inc.

Penguin Group (USA) Inc., 375 Hudson Street, New York, New York 10014, USA • Penguin Group (Canada), 90 Eglinton Avenue East, Suite 700, Toronto, Ontario M4P 2Y3, Canada (a division of Pearson Penguin Canada Inc.) • Penguin Books Ltd., 80 Strand, London WC2R 0RL, England • Penguin Ireland, 25 St. Stephen's Green, Dublin 2, Ireland (a division of Penguin Books Ltd.) • Penguin Group (Australia), 250 Camberwell Road, Camberwell, Victoria 3124, Australia (a division of Pearson Australia Group Pty. Ltd.) • Penguin Books India Pvt. Ltd., 11 Community Centre, Panchsheel Park, New Delhi—110 017, India • Penguin Group (NZ), 67 Apollo Drive, Rosedale, North Shore, Auckland 1311, New Zealand (a division of Pearson New Zealand Ltd.) • Penguin Books (South Africa) (Pty.) Ltd., 24 Sturdee Avenue, Rosebank, Johannesburg 2196, South Africa • Penguin Books Ltd., Registered Offices: 80 Strand, London WC2R 0RL, England

International Standard Book Number: 978-1-61564-699-9
Library of Congress Catalog Card Number: Available Upon Request

16 15 14   8 7 6 5 4 3 2 1

Interpretation of the printing code: The rightmost number of the first series of numbers is the year of the book's printing; the rightmost number of the second series of numbers is the number of the book's printing. For example, a printing code of 14-1 shows that the first printing occurred in 2014.

Note: This publication contains the opinions and ideas of its author. It is intended to provide helpful and informative material on the subject matter covered. It is sold with the understanding that the author and publisher are not engaged in rendering professional services in the book. If the reader requires personal assistance or advice, a competent professional should be consulted. The author and publisher specifically disclaim any responsibility for any liability, loss, or risk, personal or otherwise, which is incurred as a consequence, directly or indirectly, of the use and application of any of the contents of this book.

Most Alpha books are available at special quantity discounts for bulk purchases for sales promotions, premiums, fund-raising, or educational use. Special books, or book excerpts, can also be created to fit specific needs. For details, write: Special Markets, Alpha Books, 375 Hudson Street, New York, NY 10014.

Trademarks: All terms mentioned in this book that are known to be or are suspected of being trademarks or service marks have been appropriately capitalized. Alpha Books and Penguin Group (USA) Inc. cannot attest to the accuracy of this information. Use of a term in this book should not be regarded as affecting the validity of any trademark or service mark.

Publisher: Mike Sanders

Executive Managing Editor: Billy Fields

Senior Acquisitions Editor: Lori Cates Hand

Development Editor: Ann Barton

Production Editor: Jana M. Stefanciosa

Cover and Book Designer: Laura Merriman

Indexer: Heather McNeill

Proofreader: Jeanne Clark

CONTENTS

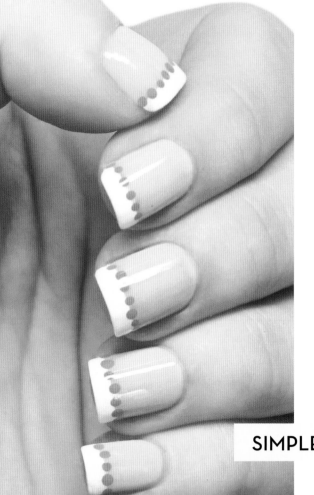

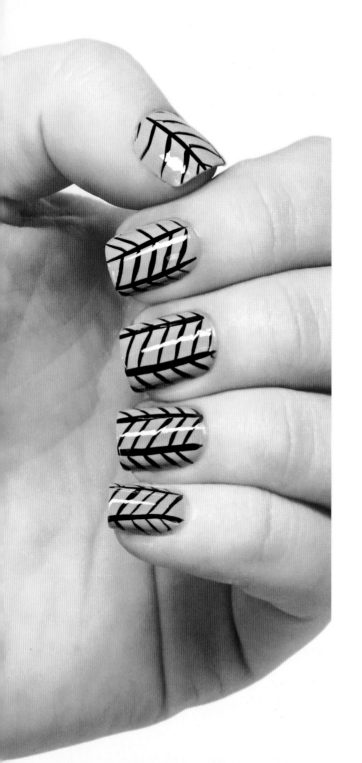

INTERMEDIATE DESIGNS 91

ADVANCED DESIGNS 149

INTRODUCTION

In today's fast-paced world, no detail goes unnoticed. That's why women and girls alike are slowing down to do their own nails in fun and bold ways. Your manicure is the finishing touch to your outfit, and there are no longer rules when it comes to colors or design. Nail art has taken the world by storm as a new way to express yourself: every style, personality, and mood can be communicated through color and art. Bold colors, graphic designs, and themed manicures are now available at most nail salons, but you can also create them on yourself and your friends at home!

Colorful manicures have been part of the world of fashion for decades. While the traditional colors and looks such as shiny red, frosty pink, and French tips are still an option, it is now appropriate to wear bold colors and graphic designs on your nails. Start simple by wearing a metallic accent nail in a shade to match your accessories. Wear bright floral nails to celebrate the start of spring, or snowflakes during the first blizzard of the season. Wear earthy, nature-inspired designs while camping or a formal glitter gradient on a date downtown. Try jack-o-lanterns for Halloween, hearts for Valentine's Day, eggs for Easter, and trees for Christmas. No matter the season or event, there is nail art that is fun and appropriate for nearly any occasion.

Manicures, pedicures, and nail art are a great way to treat yourself during a stolen moment of silence, but they can also be something fun to share with the special women in your life. Almost every woman, no matter her age or style, can appreciate pampering herself and enjoy a DIY manicure. Sisters and friends can practice their nail art skills on each other, and moms and daughters can spend quality time together over a bottle of polish. Nail parties make for great birthday parties or family gatherings! This book outlines everything you need to know to explore the world of DIY nail art, starting with nail care, proper tools for manicuring and nail art, and helpful tips and tricks in Part 1. If your nails aren't in perfect shape, you can adopt proper manicuring technique and some simple daily habits, and you will see a difference in your nails within a few weeks. Many people struggle to understand how you can create designs on such a small canvas as fingernails, but with the right tools, it can be easy. Before you get started, head to your local beauty-supply store or order the basic tools from a retailer online. Other nail services you can do at home, such as soak-off gel manicures and pedicures, are discussed in Part 1 as well.

The majority of this book features tutorials for a wide variety of nail art designs, ranging in difficulty from basic to advanced. In the simple designs in Part 2, you will learn to use some of the most important nail art tools: the dotting tool, striping brush, and striping tape, as well as a variety of items from around your home. Many of the designs in this section would be appropriate to try with younger girls who are eager to do their own nails. The intermediate and advanced designs in Parts 3 and 4 combine the basics with more intricate, freehand nail art. These tutorials take you step by step through the designs, so you will not be overwhelmed. If you are just beginning, start simple and be creative. You can switch up the designs by incorporating different colors and polish finishes. Keep practicing the simple designs until you are comfortable with your technique, and then move on to the more difficult designs. You'll be surprised at what you are capable of with a little practice!

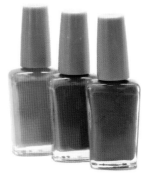

ACKNOWLEDGMENTS

Thank you to everyone who understood and supported me on this colorful journey over the past several years. To Benn, who doesn't care that our house smells like nail polish all the time, and Nance who doesn't mind that her daughter isn't a doctor. I owe a huge thanks to Debbie for all of her hard work and patience creating the images in this book. And to all of my clients, family, and friends who have shared in my excitement: I love you all!

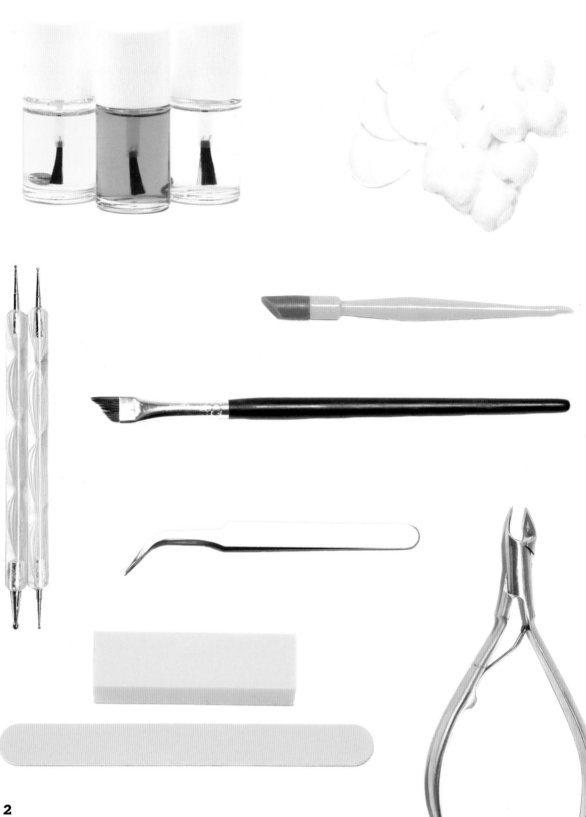

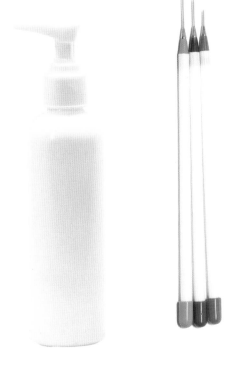

NAIL ART BASICS

Before diving into the world of nail art, it's helpful to know how to take care of your nails and hands. In this section, you will learn some essential nail care basics to turn your nails into beautiful nail art canvases. Performing a DIY manicure and polishing your nails is much more rewarding when you follow a technique that yields the best results. By using a base coat, top coat, and clean-up brush, your manicures will be clean and long-lasting. You'll also learn about other polishing options, such as soak-off gel manicures, pedicures, and toenail art.

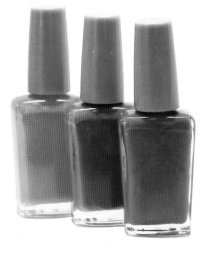

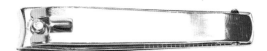

NATURAL NAIL STRUCTURE

Before you can have beautiful nails worthy of nail art, you need to understand the basic structure of your nails so you can properly care for them. The **nail plate** is the hard part of the nail that is polished. Many people probably don't think about their nails in much more detail than the nail plate, but healthy nails begin in the **nail matrix,** which is where the living, growing cells of your nails are formed. The matrix is located under your skin at the base of your nail, and sometimes can be seen showing through under the nail plate as the **lanula,** the white moon-shapes you may see at the base of your nails.

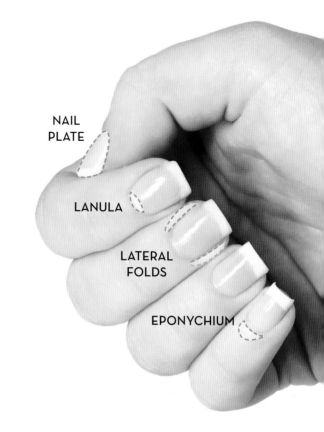

NAIL PLATE

LANULA

LATERAL FOLDS

EPONYCHIUM

In the matrix area, new nail cells are formed and pushed forward to become part of the nail plate. If your nail matrix is healthy, your nail should grow normally. The shape of your nail matrix determines how your nails grow and, therefore, the shape of your natural nail plate cannot be changed. If your nail matrix is damaged, whether from trauma or through infection, you can have permanent damage to your nails.

To protect the nail matrix and prevent entry of bacteria and other germs, the skin around your nails creates a tight seal. The sidewalls of your nails are sealed in by the **lateral folds.** Under the free edge, the **hyponychium** creates a seal between the nail bed and nail plate. The **eponychium** is the living tissue at the base of your nail that creates a seal with the nail plate. The eponychium is often referred to as the cuticle, which is incorrect terminology. The **true cuticle** is the dead, sticky tissue that grows up onto your nail plate. While the cuticle can be nipped and removed, you should never cut your eponychium.

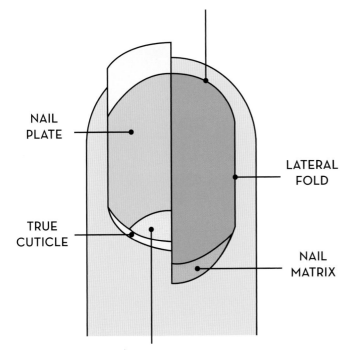

HYPONYCHIUM

NAIL
PLATE

LATERAL
FOLD

TRUE
CUTICLE

NAIL
MATRIX

LANULA

The nail plate is made up of about 100 layers of nail cells and keratin, the same protein that makes up the skin and hair. The keratin proteins are connected together by cross-links, which help to create the tough, hard structure of the nail plate. There are small spaces or channels between the keratin layers that usually contain water and oil. The water/oil balance in the nail plate helps determine the health of the nail. Dry nails are more rigid and more likely to break. Too much water can cause your nail to expand or become flimsy. Limiting overexposure to water and using cuticle oils on your nails can help maintain this moisture balance and create a healthy, balanced nail.

In the coming pages, you will learn how to best care for your nails through day-to-day behaviors and maintenance through manicures.

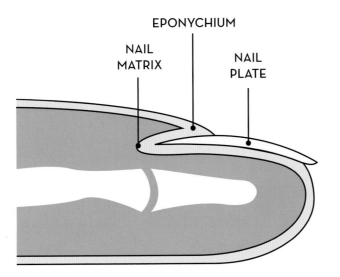

EPONYCHIUM

NAIL
MATRIX

NAIL
PLATE

MANICURE PRODUCTS

To maintain healthy and beautiful nails, you need to perform regular manicures and do some daily maintenance using the products shown here.

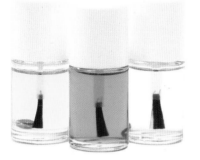

BASE COAT, TOP COAT, AND CUTICLE OIL

A complete manicure includes all three of these products and, without them, your polish will chip quickly and appear dull. Base coat protects your nails from staining and helps polish adhere to the nail plate. Top coat creates a shiny surface, and some formulations even help speed up dry time. Cuticle oil is necessary for healthy, soft skin around your nail plate and should be used regularly, both during manicures and during daily nail maintenance.

NAIL TREATMENTS

Nail treatments are similar to a base coat but are specially formulated with proteins and different chemicals to promote strong nails.

CLEAN-UP BRUSH

Even professionals sometimes make mistakes. An inexpensive angled eyeliner brush dipped in acetone can be used to clean polish off of the skin and cuticle. This is especially helpful in messy nail art techniques!

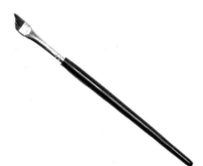

COTTON

Cotton balls or lint-free cotton pads are a staple on any manicure table. Cotton can be used to remove polish or apply product to the fingers.

CUTICLE REMOVER

Cuticle removers are creams or gels that dissolve dead tissue from your nail plate. With regular use, your cuticles will be manageable and your nails will appear clean and smooth.

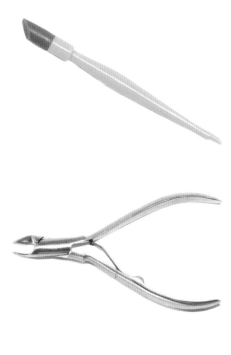

CUTICLE PUSHER

Cuticle pushers come in many forms, but for the DIY manicurist, a soft plastic one is best. This tool is used to gently scrape dead cuticle tissue off the nail plate and carefully push back the eponychium. Metal cuticle pushers and disposable wooden sticks can also be used for this purpose, but should be used with caution.

CUTICLE NIPPERS

Cuticle nippers are used to cut dead tissue from the nail plate. Nippers should not be used to cut the living eponychium. Sticky cuticle tissue that cannot be removed with a cuticle pusher can be cut from the nail plate, and hangnails can be carefully nipped to avoid ripping.

NAIL CLIPPERS

Nail clippers are used to trim the free edge of the nails. These should be used when the length being removed is too great for filing to be convenient.

FILES AND BUFFERS

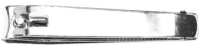

Nail files are used to shape and remove length from natural nails. On most people, a file with a 240 grit works best, as it will not be too rough for soft natural nails. Buffers are used to smooth the nail plate of ridges and prep for nail enhancements. Buffing should be done with caution.

HAND CREAM

Hand creams and lotions are used to moisturize the hands and arms. Moisturized hands are healthier and younger looking.

NAIL ART TOOLS

Many people struggle with creating beautiful nail art because they lack the proper tools. For the tutorials in this book, you will need a few industry-specific tools as well as some common household items. You can find these tools at beauty supply stores or online.

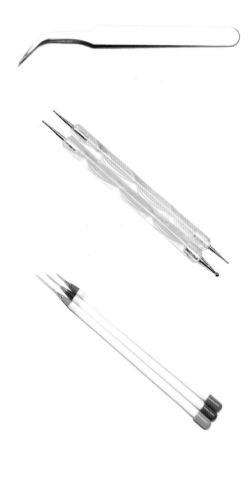

NAIL ART TWEEZERS

These tweezers have a specialized shape that makes it easy to place elements onto the nails or remove fuzz or imperfections from freshly polished nails. Regular tweezers can work as well.

DOTTING TOOLS

The dotting tool is the most basic nail art tool, and it can be used to create a wide variety of designs such as polka dots, leopard print, and flowers. Most dotting tools are double-ended and vary in size. A dotting tool with one large end and one small end works best, but they often come in five-packs, ensuring you will have all the sizes you need. There are also some everyday items that can be used to create dots: the rounded end of a bobby pin or the head of a pin stuck into a wine cork are affordable, DIY options. To use a dotting tool, simply dip the end into a puddle of polish and press it gently against the nail plate.

STRIPING BRUSHES

These long, thin brushes work best for making lines and small details. While any small paintbrushes can work, affordable striping brushes are available at beauty supply stores and online.

POLISH PALETTE

When you use dotting tools and striping brushes, you need to dip your tool into a small puddle of polish. You can use a paint palette from the store for this purpose, but a paper plate, index card, or piece of aluminum foil will work just as well. Simply use the polish brush to drop a small amount of polish onto your palette, and you are ready to create.

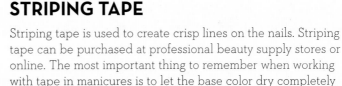

STRIPING TAPE

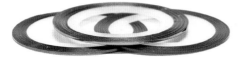

Striping tape is used to create crisp lines on the nails. Striping tape can be purchased at professional beauty supply stores or online. The most important thing to remember when working with tape in manicures is to let the base color dry completely before applying the tape.

STUDS, STONES, GLITTER, AND FOILS

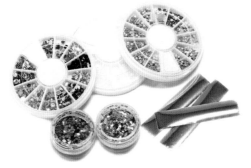

A wide variety of elements can be applied to your nails. Studs, rhinestones, nail charms, and loose glitter can be purchased at beauty supply stores and online, as well as at general craft stores. While these products are designed for use on the nail, there are many other things that you could adhere to your nail plate. If you like a bold, wild look, keep an eye open for small trinkets that could become makeshift nail charms!

Nail foils are metallic foil strips with a clear backing, to make them easy to apply to the nail. They are available in solid colors and designs. While there are a variety of ways to use foils, you must use a foil adhesive if you want to apply the foils smoothly to the entire nail.

ACRYLIC PAINT

For detail-oriented artists, acrylic paint may work better than traditional nail polish. Although it is not designed specifically for nail art, acrylic paint is water-soluble and safe to use on nails. It dries quickly, stays where you put it, and becomes shiny when finished with a top coat. Affordable acrylic paints can be purchased at any craft store.

HOUSEHOLD ITEMS

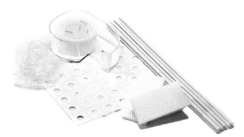

Many of the tools used in the tutorials in this book you probably already have in your home: straws, cosmetic sponges, plastic wrap, hole-punch stickers, and stationery tape.

MANICURING BASICS

The perfect nail art manicure looks its best when it starts with healthy and well-maintained nails. By implementing a few simple habits into your daily routine and adopting healthy manicure techniques, you will see a difference in your nails in just a few days. Perform an at-home manicure biweekly to stay on top of your nail care routine and create strong, beautiful nails.

MATERIALS

- Nail file
- Cuticle remover
- Cuticle pusher
- Cuticle oil
- Hand cream
- Cotton balls
- Nail polish remover or acetone
- Nail treatment
- Base coat
- Nail polish
- Top coat
- Clean-up brush

1

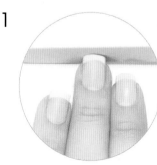

File your nails to desired length and shape. File in one direction at a time, avoiding a sawing motion. Always use a gentle, high-grit file on natural nails.

2

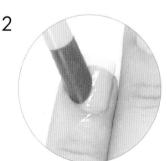

Apply a cuticle remover to your nail plate. Using a cuticle pusher, gently push back your cuticles. Do not push too hard or force the eponychium back. Only if needed, use nippers to remove only the sticky cuticle tissue that may be stuck to the nail plate. Never cut your eponychium, as this is living tissue.

3

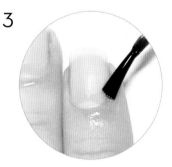

Apply a cuticle oil to your eponychium and massage into your nail plate and fingertip. Caring for your eponychium is crucial to healthy nail growth and a clean, finished manicure.

4

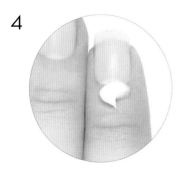

Apply hand cream to your hands, taking time to massage it into your nail plate.

5

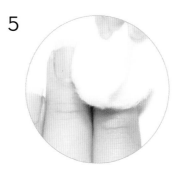

Remove all oil and debris from your nail plate using a cotton ball soaked in acetone or polish remover. This will help the polish adhere to your nail properly.

6

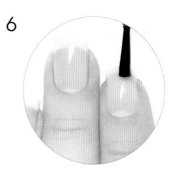

If needed, apply a nail treatment to your clean nail plate. While most nail treatments can also function as a base coat, I like to use both products in my manicures. Base coat helps prevent staining and helps your polish adhere to your nail plate.

7

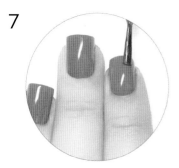

Polish your nails with the color of your choice as outlined in Polishing Basics.

8

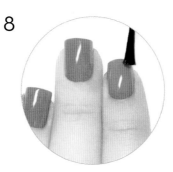

Always finish your manicure with a fast-dry top coat. This not only helps dry your polish, but it also creates a shiny, long-lasting finish.

9

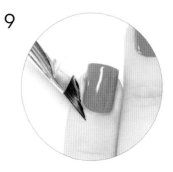

If needed, clean excess polish off your eponychium and fingers using an angled eyeliner brush dipped in acetone polish remover.

POLISHING BASICS

Polishing your nails does not need to be a stressful experience. Once you have practiced proper polishing technique, you will find this ritual relaxing and enjoyable! Follow these steps on well-manicured nails to create a long-lasting, beautiful base for your nail art. When following the tutorials outlined in this book, always use base coat, top coat, and the clean-up technique outlined here.

MATERIALS

- Base coat
- Nail polish
- Top coat
- Clean-up brush
- Acetone

The most difficult part of polishing your own nails at home is polishing your dominant hand on your own. Some people are more ambidextrous than others, but with plenty of practice your weak hand will become stronger. Rest your elbow and forearm on a table to steady your hand when polishing your dominant hand, and always remember that you can use a clean-up brush to fix mistakes if you get shaky.

1

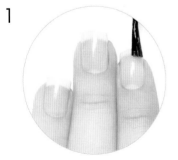

Apply base coat to each nail, covering the entire nail plate. Let dry.

2

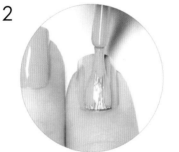

Press the polish brush against your nail plate, pushing it down as close to the cuticle as possible without touching it. Repeat if needed to get closer to the eponychium.

3

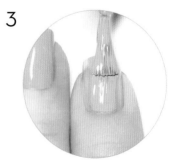

Pull the brush toward the free edge of the nail, creating a stroke of polish.

4

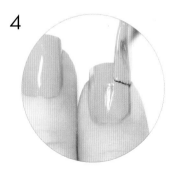

Using a similar method, apply a brush stroke to the right side of your nail.

5

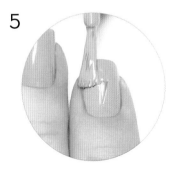

Repeat step 4 on the left side of your nail plate.

6

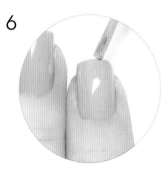

Gently run the brush along the free edge of your nail, sealing the tip of your nail plate.

7

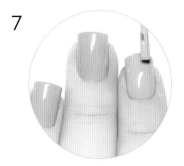

Repeat steps 2 through 6 with a second coat of polish.

8

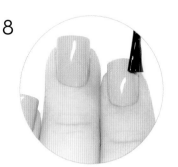

Apply top coat with a full brush and a light hand.

9

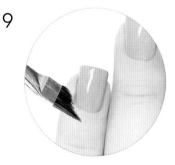

Use an angled eyeliner brush dipped in acetone to clean up excess polish on your skin or cuticle. This is a great tip for beginners and experienced polishers alike.

GOOD NAIL HABITS

Regular manicures are very important for beautiful nails, but if you completely ignore your hands and nails between manicures, you will not see long-term improvement in your nails' appearance and health. A few simple daily habits can make a big difference in your nails.

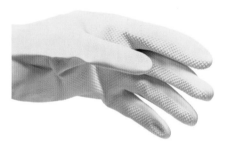

PROTECT YOUR HANDS

Exposure to water and chemicals can damage your nails and cause your manicure to chip and dull. If you can, avoid soaking your nails for long periods while bathing and swimming, and wear rubber gloves while doing dishes, cleaning, or handling household chemicals. This will not only protect your nails, but will also help keep your skin away from potentially harmful solvents and detergents.

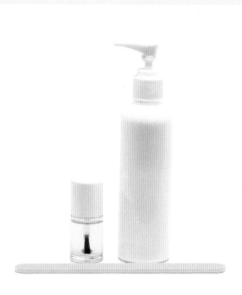

DAILY MAINTENANCE

Daily nail maintenance is a simple way to keep your nails in shape between manicures. When you apply hand cream, take a few extra seconds to massage it into your eponychium and apply cuticle oil or balm at least once each day. Keeping your nails well-oiled helps to maintain a healthy moisture balance, which leads to more flexible, chip- and tear-resistant nail plates. Cuticle oils and balms can also encourage healthy nail growth and extend the life of your manicure.

When performing your at-home manicure, there are some other habits to keep in mind. Rough filing in a sawing motion can shear apart layers of your nail, leading to peeling. Always file your nails from the outside corners to the center of the free edge, in one direction at a time. Also, when dealing with your cuticles and eponychium, be extremely cautious. The eponychium should not be cut or pushed back with force, as this can lead to nail matrix damage.

AVOID

- Excessive soaking in water
- Exposure to chemicals
- Filing with a sawing motion
- Using your nails as tools
- Excessive buffing
- Cutting the eponychium

ALWAYS

- Apply cuticle oil daily.
- Keep hands moisturized.
- Wear rubber gloves.
- File in one direction at a time.

PRODUCT INGREDIENTS

Many of the qualities we look for in nail polishes—rich color, shiny finish, smooth consistency—are achieved thanks to the chemicals used in the polish formulas. Although these chemicals optimize performance, some of them have been shown to have health risks. There are many options on the market now, allowing consumers to make their own decisions about chemical exposure. This is a personal decision, but it is best to be educated on these ingredients, regardless of what choices you make.

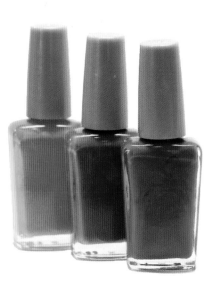

THE BIG THREE

Formaldehyde, toluene, and dibutyl phthalate (DBP) are commonly referred to as the "Big 3," a group of chemicals known to cause harmful effects such as cancer or birth defects. In the past these ingredients were used in many polishes, but now many companies exclude them from their formulations. Polishes referred to as "3-free" do not contain these potentially harmful chemicals. Most brands available in salons or the drug store are now 3-free. Always check the ingredient list on the bottle or label to be sure. Pregnant women and children should avoid using polishes and products that are not 3-free.

Some companies offer "5-free" polishes, meaning they do not contain the Big 3 or formaldehyde resin and camphor, which are other potential irritants. 5-free companies include Zoya, Priti NYC, SpaRitual, Chanel, and other boutique brands.

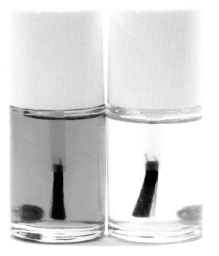

TOP COAT AND NAIL TREATMENT INGREDIENTS

There are a wide variety of top coats on the market, some containing the Big 3 chemicals. Top coats that contain DBP or toluene, referred to as 2-free, are thicker, so they create an ultra-smooth, shiny finish for your manicure. They also tend to perform better over nail art, as smearing is minimal. 3-free top coats are thinner, but still dry to a shiny finish. You may need to wait for your nail art to dry completely and then apply multiple coats to achieve a completely smooth surface. No matter which choice you make, it is important to understand the pros and cons of each product and its ingredient list.

Similar to top coats, there are nail treatments on the market that contain formaldehyde. Formaldehyde helps to create more cross-links between the layers of your nails, making your nails stronger, but over time, exposure to formaldehyde can make your nails brittle. Formaldehyde nail treatments work well for many people, but if you prefer to use a formaldehyde-free option, those are readily available as well.

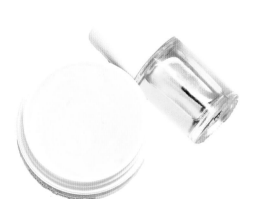

CREAM AND TREATMENT INGREDIENTS

Hand creams, cuticle oils, and cuticle balms also contain a wide variety of ingredients that should be understood. Natural oils and butters are a great choice since they are most similar to the natural oils your body produces. Jojoba oil is molecularly small enough to penetrate the nail plate, leading to a healthy moisture balance and increased flexibility. Shea butter has great healing qualities that are good for your skin. When purchasing products you may also want to consider whether the product is tested on animals, paraben-free, vegan, gluten-free, or organic.

GEL MANICURES

The nail industry is always changing as companies develop new product lines and innovations. Recently, the industry has been moving in the direction of soak-off gel manicures. Gel manicures are longer lasting than traditional manicures. Many brands boast up to two weeks of shiny color. You don't have to go to a nail salon for a gel manicure; there are many kits available that you can purchase at a drug store or online and do at home. The basics of an at-home gel manicure are covered here, but it is imperative that you follow the directions and use the products provided in the gel manicure kit that you purchase.

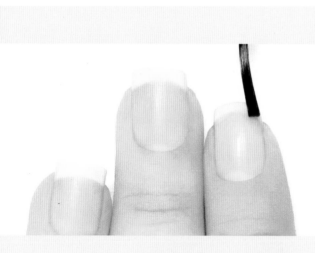

PREPARING FOR THE MANICURE

Gel manicures start with the same preparation work as a regular manicure: gently push your eponychium back, clean your nails of excess cuticle tissue, and shape your free edge. Clean your nail plates with polish remover or isopropyl alcohol.

For the gel polish to adhere to the nail plate properly, you need to dehydrate your nail plate. Most brands have a dehydrator that is optimized to work with their system. The dehydrator shown here uses a brush-on formula. Some kits will instruct you to also buff your nail plate to remove shine; if so, do this with caution.

Gel polishes are generally thicker than regular polish, so there is a learning curve when you begin working with them. Apply thin coats to prevent bubbles or lifting.

All gel manicure kits are different. Some require base coat and top coat, while others have a 3-in-1 formulation. Whatever kit you choose, be sure to follow the application and removal directions closely for best results.

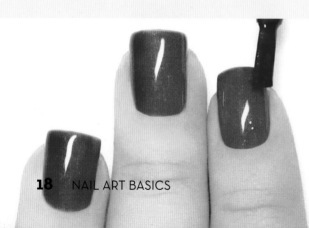

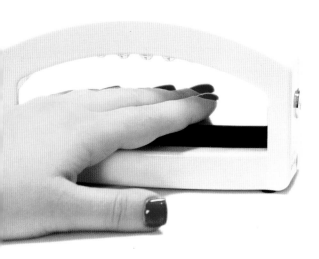

CURING THE GEL MANICURE

The biggest investment in doing gel manicures at home is a UV or LED lamp. Gel polishes require UV or LED to start the polymerization, or curing of the product. Without a lamp, your manicure will never dry. UV lamps are generally more affordable, but take two minutes, on average, to cure one coat of gel polish. LED lamps are more expensive, but they take only 30 seconds to cure a layer of polish, and the bulbs do not need to be replaced as often as UV lamps. Most gel manicure kits available at drug stores and beauty supply stores come with a small lamp that is optimized to work with that specific system.

DOING NAIL ART WITH GEL POLISH

Nail art can be done using gel polish as well. Be sure to remember to cure each color you apply before layering something over it. Tape manicures are especially convenient with gel manicures because the polish is completely dry once it has been cured, eliminating dry time.

3D ELEMENTS

3D elements can create a wide variety of manicures. Girly and feminine or edgy and bold, you can achieve nearly any look using 3D elements. Since this style of manicure does not require any freehand skill, it is a great way to start with nail art!

Whether you are working with nail studs or rhinestones, loose glitter, or nail charms, the application is similar. Depending on how long you want your manicure to last, you can apply elements using just top coat, or using a nail adhesive or glue.

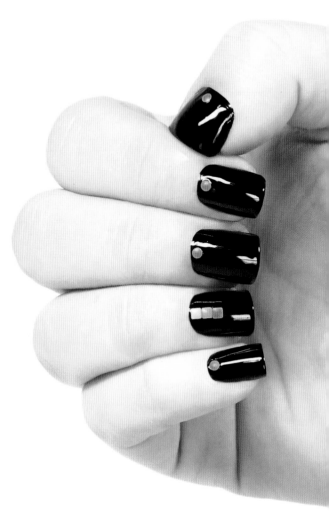

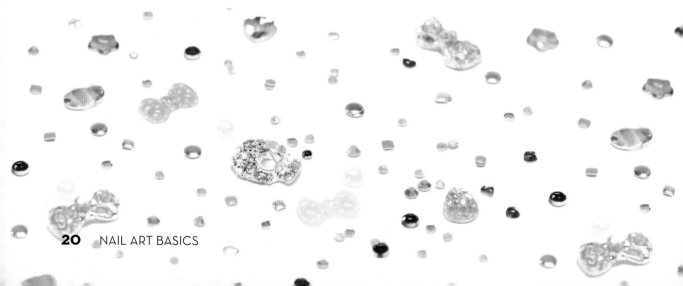

NAIL GLUE

To apply 3D elements to your nails for extended wear, apply a drop of nail glue or adhesive to a dry manicure. Use nail art tweezers to place the 3D element in the drop of adhesive. Hold in place until the adhesive begins to dry. If desired, you can apply a layer of thick top coat over small 3D elements, such as studs or rhinestones, for added hold. Nail glue or adhesive generally requires acetone soaking for removal.

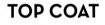

TOP COAT

For a gentler option, you can apply 3D elements using top coat. This works best with smaller elements such as studs, rhinestones, loose glitter, and small charms. Let your manicure dry completely and then apply a layer of top coat. Use nail art tweezers to apply your 3D elements onto the wet top coat and let dry. Seal everything in with a coat of thick top coat for added hold. Generally, small 3D elements applied this way will last for a few days with regular wear.

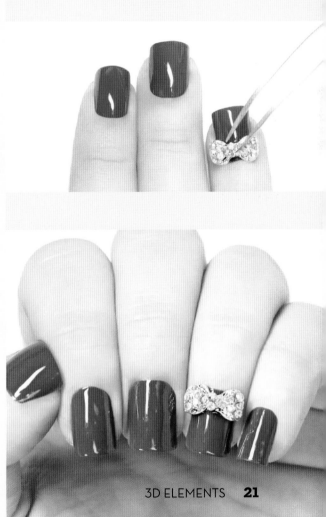

POLISH REMOVAL

Regular nail polish can be easily removed with nail polish remover. Acetone is a solvent commonly used in nail salons because of its effectiveness. Acetone works quickly to dissolve the polish and remove it from your nails and skin, which limits the amount of time you are exposed to it. However, acetone also has strong fumes that can lead to headaches and dizziness with overexposure. Non-acetone polish removers are also available, as well as moisturizing acetone-based formulas that are less harsh. While non-acetone removers may seem safer, they still contain chemical solvents, so they should not be overused.

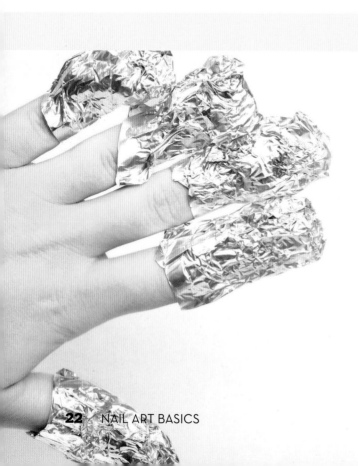

THE FOIL METHOD

For gel manicures or tough-to-remove glitter polishes, the foil method is a great option. Simply soak a cotton ball in pure acetone and place it directly on the nail plate. Wrap your entire fingertip in a piece of foil. This will hold the solvent to your nail and prevent it from evaporating. Allow this to sit for about 5 minutes for a glitter manicure or 15 minutes for a gel manicure. The polish should slide right off your nail when you pull the foil off. For gel manicures, if 15 minutes was not long enough, apply a fresh acetone-soaked cotton ball and rewrap for an additional five minutes. Repeat until the gel polish lifts from the nail plate.

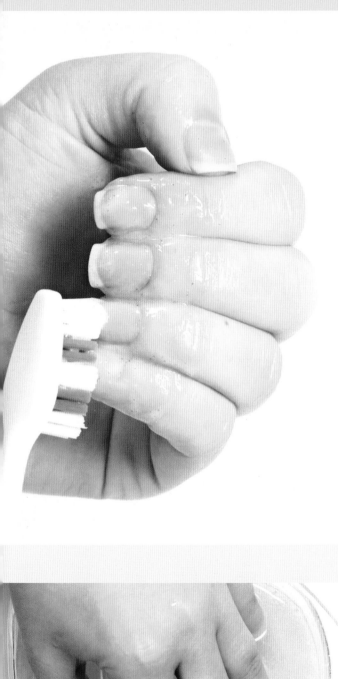

STAIN REMOVAL

When polishing your nails, staining can occur. There are a variety of products on the market that help to remove these, as well as some easy at-home remedies. Certain shades of polish are notorious for staining, especially bold blues and greens.

If you remove your polish to find your nail plates tinted, the first approach to try is scrubbing with whitening toothpaste. The same ingredients that remove stains from your teeth can remove fresh stains from your nails. You can also scrub with a baking-soda-and-water paste. Keep an old toothbrush specifically for this purpose.

Older, hard-to-remove stains may require more than a simple scrub. Whitening soaks are available at most beauty supply stores, or you can create your own soak with lemon juice and water. Before soaking, gently buff your nails using a high-grit buffer to remove some of the surface staining. 2400 grit works well on healthy natural nails. Add several drops of lemon juice to warm water in a bowl or manicure dish and soak for 10 to 15 minutes. For store-bought whitening soaks, always follow the instructions on the package.

PEDICURES AND TOENAIL ART

Just as manicuring is the art of caring for and beautifying the hands, a pedicure takes care of the feet. Pedicures are luxurious and can be extremely relaxing. Toenails and feet are cared for similarly to fingernails and hands, with a few additions to aid in the removal of rough skin on the feet. While pedicures are generally a salon or spa service, you can easily perform one on yourself at home.

SOAKING

Pedicures begin with the soaking of the feet. This helps to soften the skin and cuticles and is extremely relaxing. Fill a large bowl (or the bathtub) with warm water and add a foot soak or bath salts. Soak your feet for at least 10 minutes. Remove your feet from the water and pat dry.

NAIL CARE

The basic pedicure procedure involves shaping the toenails and caring for the cuticles just like you would do in a manicure. Toenails should be clipped and filed as straight across as possible to avoid ingrown nails. Once the nails and cuticles are in good shape, you are ready to take care of the rest of your feet.

SCRUBS

Pedicure scrubs contain sugar, salt, or other exfoliates to help remove rough, dead skin. Apply a liberal amount of scrub to your feet and massage it in with damp hands, focusing on the heels and balls of your feet. If desired, use a foot file or pumice stone to smooth the roughest areas. When finished, rinse the scrub from your feet with warm water and pat dry.

MOISTURIZING

Moisturizing your skin is crucial on all parts of your body, including your feet. Massage a thick cream into your feet, again focusing on the dry areas as well as the cuticles and tips of the toes. This should be done daily to maintain soft feet. Remove the lotion from the nail plate using a cotton ball and polish remover to prep your toenails for polish. Always use a base coat, top coat, and proper cleanup technique when polishing your toenails.

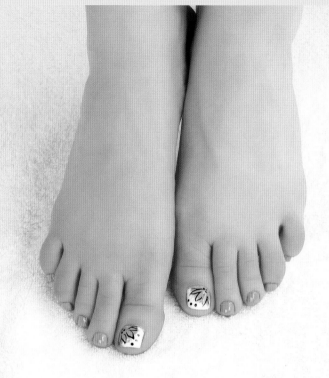

NAIL ART FOR YOUR TOES

Many of the nail art designs in this book can be adapted for the toenails with a bit of creativity. For some designs, it works best to feature the pattern on the big toe and polish the other toenails in a coordinating solid color, as shown in the Splash Floral pedicure.

For other designs, all five nails can feature nail art, though it may be difficult to fit detailed patterns on small toenails. The Leopard I design makes for a great eye-catching pedicure. Polka dots, florals, and animal print designs are the most popular choices for toenails, but the possibilities are truly endless.

Splash Floral

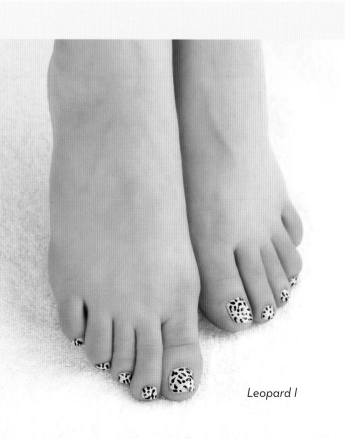

Leopard I

COMBINING TECHNIQUES

This book features 77 nail art designs, but there are literally thousands of possibilities within these pages. By changing the colors or polish finishes used in the tutorials, you can change the entire look of a design and make it appropriate for nearly any event or occasion. You can also combine designs to create unique manicures by layering different elements together or painting different designs on each nail.

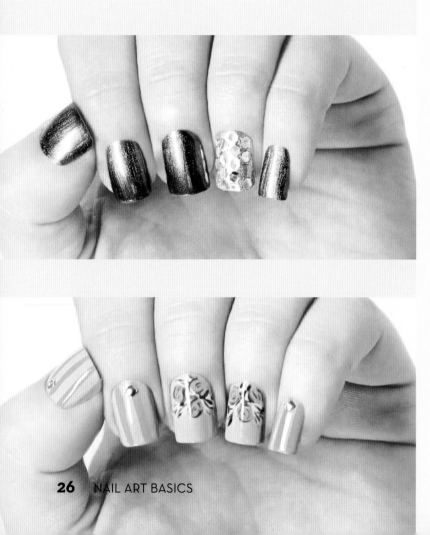

THE ACCENT NAIL

The simplest way to put two designs together is with an accent nail or two. This refers to one or two nails that are polished differently than the others and is usually done on the ring finger or middle finger. Commonly, an accent nail of nail art is paired with a coordinating solid color on the other nails, but two nail art designs could be used as well. Here, a disco ball accent nail pops against a solid blue manicure.

Vertical stripes, nail studs, and detailed roses come together in this beautiful double accent nail manicure. The two designs are nothing alike, but when done in the same color family, they create a cohesive look.

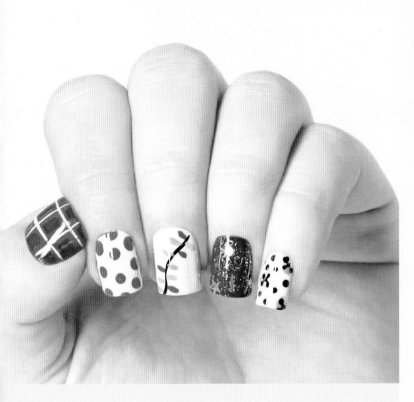

SKITTLE MANICURES

When a manicure features a different design on each nail in a similar color family or theme, it is referred to as a "skittle" manicure. The holiday skittle manicure featured here includes multiple Christmas-themed designs and polishes. Other variations of a skittle manicure include one design done in five different color schemes or five separate designs done in the same color scheme.

LAYERING

Some of the nail art designs covered in this book lend themselves to layering. Gradients, plastic wrap texture, and dry brushing are great bases for nail art such as black leopard print, zebra stripes, or a striping tape manicure. Some of the tutorials in this book combine these techniques, but be creative and you will come up with some unique manicures, like the gradient and leopard print design shown here.

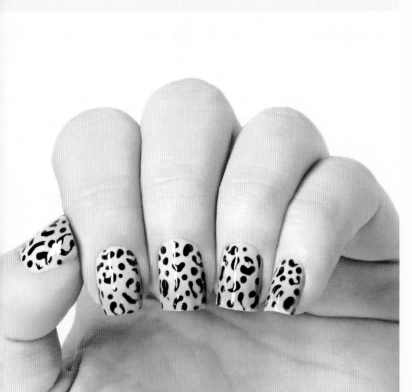

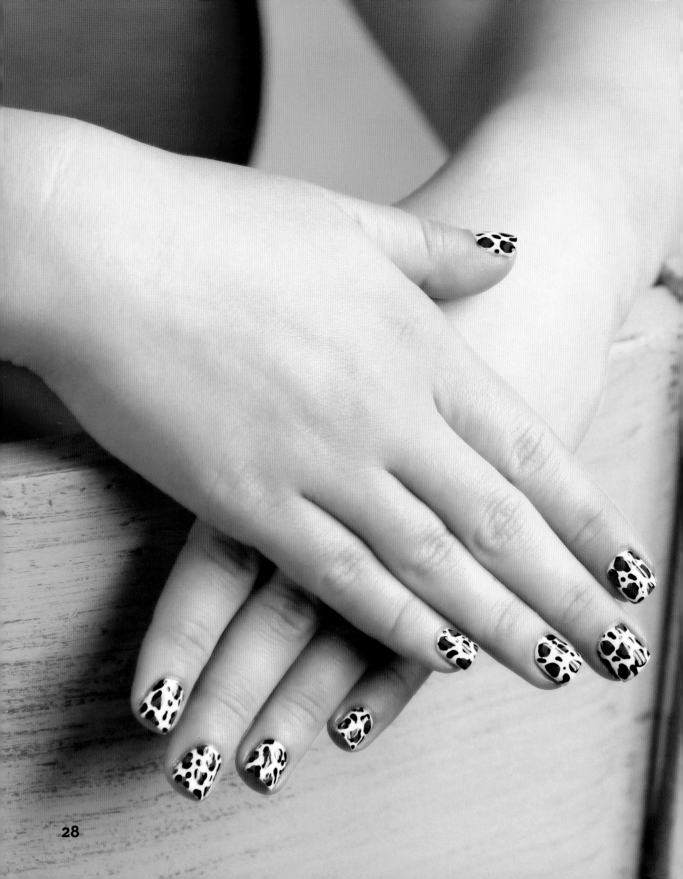

SIMPLE
DESIGNS

There are countless nail art designs that can be created using a few basic tools: striping brushes, dotting tools, and tape. Even beginning nail artists can find success with polka dots and stripes! This section covers 30 manicures that use these basic tools, as well as a few common household items. Practice and master the techniques in this section, and you will be well prepared to move on to more complex designs.

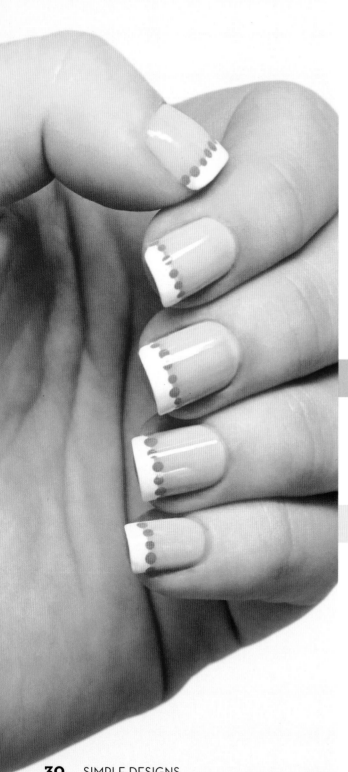

DOTTY FRENCH

Perhaps the most classic of all nail art techniques is the French tip. It's perfect for formal occasions in its original form, but with a few polka dots, it becomes a fun manicure that can be worn anytime. Using tape will help you achieve a perfect edge.

MATERIALS

• Tape
• Dotting tool
• Polish palette

POLISH COLORS

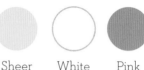

Sheer pink   White   Pink

1

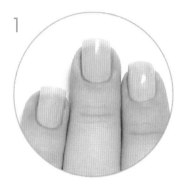

Polish your nails in a sheer pink shade and allow to dry completely.

2

TAPE

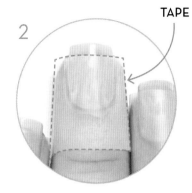

Apply a piece of stationery tape to each nail, leaving the very tip of the nail exposed.

3

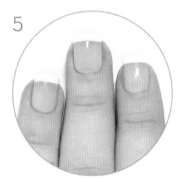

On just one nail, apply a white polish where the nail is exposed, creating the French tip.

4

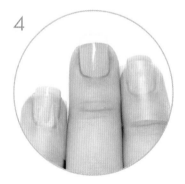

Immediately after applying the white tip, carefully remove the tape from the nail.

5

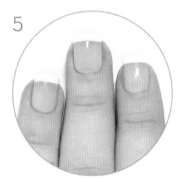

Follow steps 3 and 4 to create white tips on the rest of your nails.

6

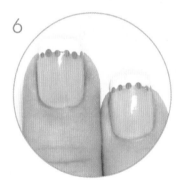

Dip your dotting tool into a puddle of pink polish and make dots along the line where the sheer pink and white polishes meet.

CLASSIC DOTTICURE

Polka-dot manicures can be girly, classic, or edgy, depending on the color palette you choose. Using a dotting tool, dots are easy to create and master. A simple black and white color scheme creates a look that is perfect any time of year.

MATERIALS

• Dotting tool
• Polish palette

POLISH COLORS

Black   White

1

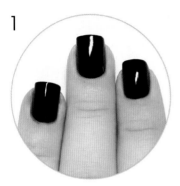

Polish your nails with black polish.

2

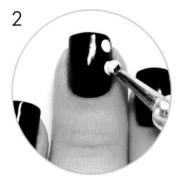

Dip your dotting tool into a small pool of white polish. With gentle pressure, press the dotting tool against your nail to create a dot.

3

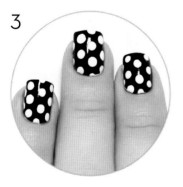

Continue creating dots on all nails in a staggered pattern.

The dotting tool is one of the most versatile nail art tools. In a simple dotticure, your dots can be staggered, set in a line, or randomly placed around the nail. Once you are comfortable with basic dots, there are many other designs you can create using just your dotting tool, including leopard print and floral patterns.

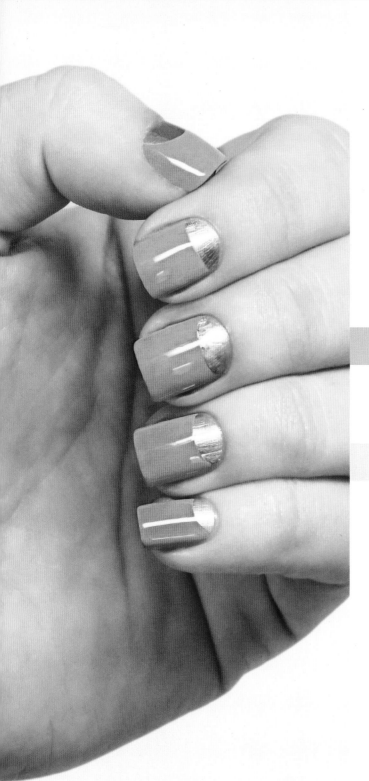

HALF-MOONS

A truly vintage design, the half-moon manicure is extremely versatile. Use contrasting colors or finishes to create something subtle or flashy on your fingertips.

MATERIALS

• Hole-punch reinforcement stickers
• Scissors

POLISH COLORS

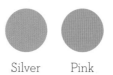

Silver Pink

1

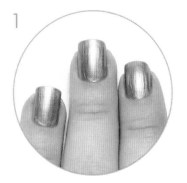

Polish your nail in the color you want your half-moon to be. Here, it will be metallic silver.

Use scissors to snip open each hole-punch reinforcement sticker. This makes them easier to work with.

2

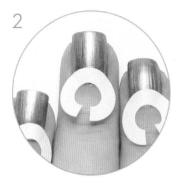

Once the silver polish is dry, apply a sticker to the base of each nail, covering a "moon" shape.

3

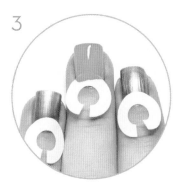

Carefully polish one nail with pink polish.

4

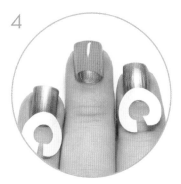

Immediately after polishing your nail, carefully remove the hole-punch sticker.

5

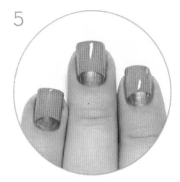

Repeat steps 4 and 5 on the rest of your nails, completing the half-moon manicure.

LEOPARD I

Leopard print is the perfect design to bring out your sassy side! Once you have mastered dots with your dotting tool, leopard print is an easy next step. Whether you use funky bright colors or traditional earth tones, the finished product always is eye-catching.

MATERIALS

• Dotting tool
• Polish palette

POLISH COLORS

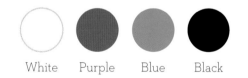

White   Purple   Blue   Black

1

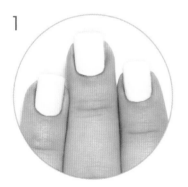

Polish your nails with white polish. Let dry for a few minutes.

2

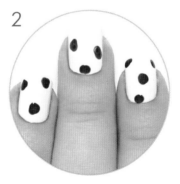

Use your dotting tool to apply a few small "spots" in purple on each nail. They should be irregularly shaped, not perfectly round.

3

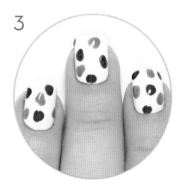

Using the same technique, apply some blue spots. Space them randomly on the nail.

4

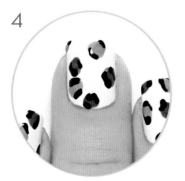

Use your dotting tool to create the black detailing on each spot. C-shapes work well.

5

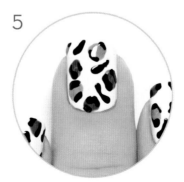

Using gentle pressure and your dotting tool, create a few curved black lines between the colored spots.

6

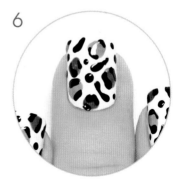

Fill in any empty space with small black dots.

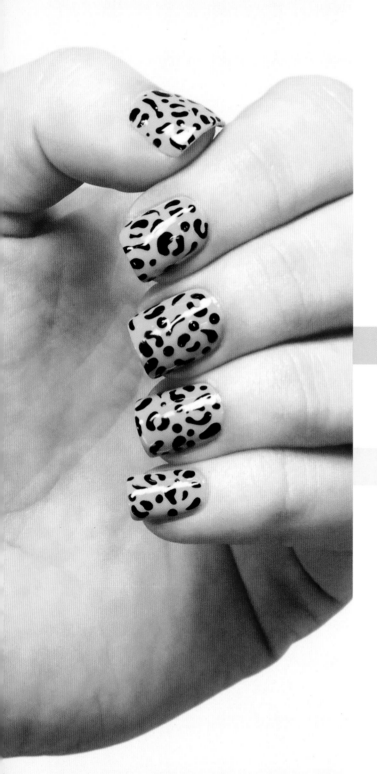

LEOPARD II

Leopard print can be produced in several ways. With this technique, you create the print using only black polish, so you can apply it over a variety of bases: solid colors, gradients, or other textures. The only limit to what you can do is your creativity!

MATERIALS

• Dotting tool
• Polish palette

POLISH COLORS

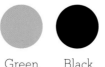

Green   Black

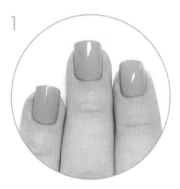

1

Polish your nails in your base color—in this example, a funky bright green. Let dry for a few minutes.

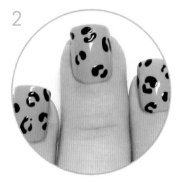

2

Using a small dotting tool, create leopard spots on your nails in black polish. C-shapes work well.

Leopard print isn't perfect in nature, and it doesn't need to be perfect on your nail. Your leopard spots can be U-shaped, pairs of C-shapes, or even full circles. Experiment with what you like best. Keep your dotting tool covered in polish and use a light pressure when touching the tool to your nail with smooth, sweeping motions.

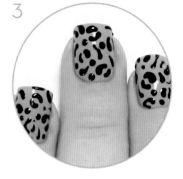

3

Using a light pressure with your dotting tool, create curved black lines and dots to fill the nail.

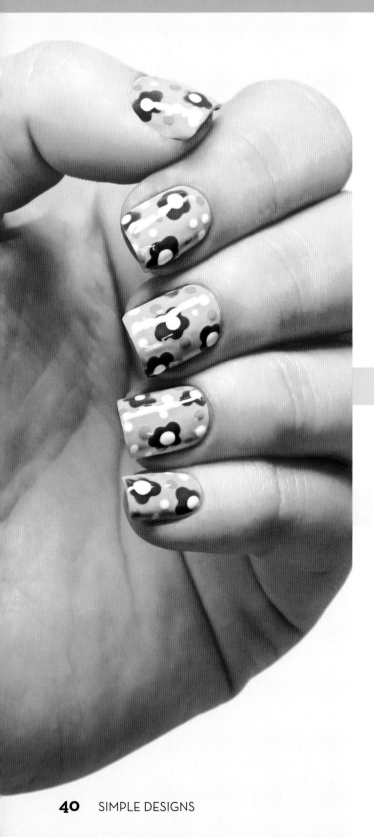

RETRO FLORAL

The Retro Floral is one of the easiest floral nail art designs to master. Using only your dotting tool, you can create a fun yet whimsical manicure suitable for all young souls, regardless of age.

MATERIALS

• Dotting tool
• Polish palette

POLISH COLORS

Blue   Purple   White   Green

1

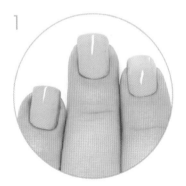

Polish your nails light blue.

2

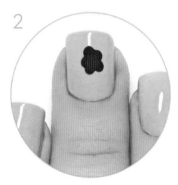

Using your dotting tool, make five overlapping purple dots in a circular shape. This should resemble a flower.

3

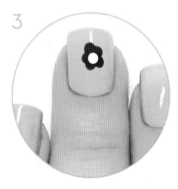

Place a white dot in the center of the flower shape.

4

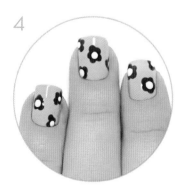

Repeat steps 2 and 3, filling each nail with flowers. Create an all-over print by placing parts of flowers over the edge of your nails.

5

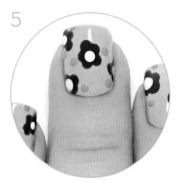

Using the small end of your dotting tool, place one or two green dots near each flower.

6

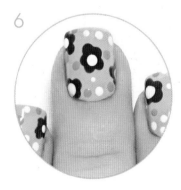

Fill any remaining space with small white dots.

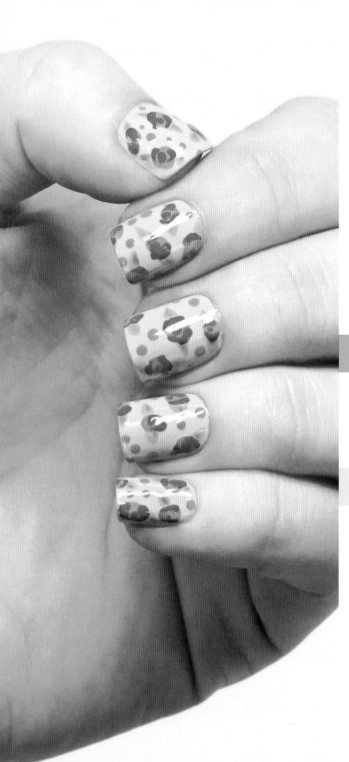

VINTAGE ROSES

Floral prints are the epitome of classy nail art manicures. This vintage rose design appears more difficult than it is. Shades of pink and green add depth to this sophisticated yet simple design.

MATERIALS

- Dotting tool
- Polish palette
- Striping brush

POLISH COLORS

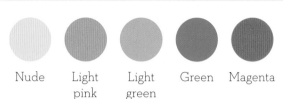

Nude   Light pink   Light green   Green   Magenta

1

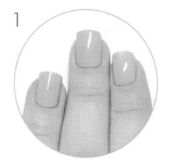

Polish your nails in a nude shade. Choose a neutral that complements your skin tone. Allow to dry.

2

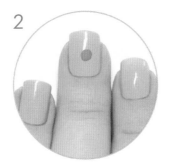

Using your dotting tool, create a round light pink shape on your nail. This will become a rose.

3

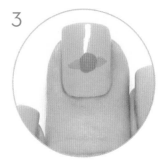

Use your striping brush to draw a light green triangle on either side of the circle.

4

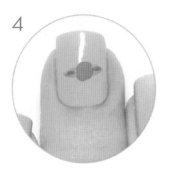

Add a dark green detail line down the center of each triangle, using your striping brush. These are the leaves.

5

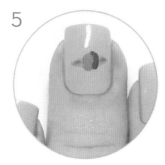

Use the small end of your dotting tool to add a magenta C-shape on one side of the circle.

6

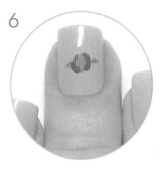

Add a magenta C-shape on the other side of the rose. This should cover where the leaves meet the rose.

7

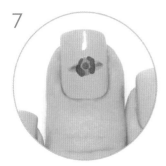

Place a small magenta dot in the middle of the circle, finishing the rose.

8

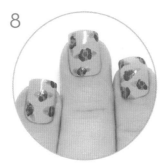

Repeat steps 2 through 7, spacing the roses out over all of your nails.

9

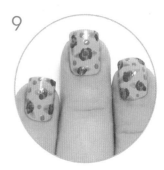

Add several green or pink dots around the flowers to fill any empty space on the nail.

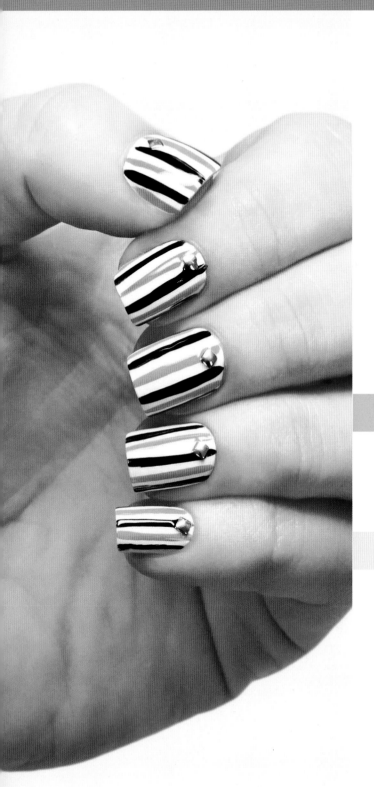

VERTICAL STRIPES

Aside from dots, stripes are one of the most basic nail art elements. On their own or as a part of a more complex manicure, stripes are graphic and eye-catching. A striping brush or long, thin paint brush works best for this technique.

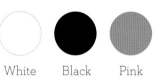

1

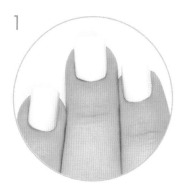

Polish your nails with white polish. Place a puddle of black polish on your palette and load your striping brush.

2

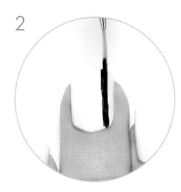

Allow the brush to make contact with your nail near the cuticle and gently pull toward the free edge.

3

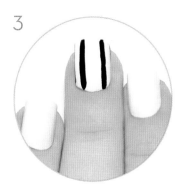

Add one or two more black stripes, spacing them out evenly over your nail.

4

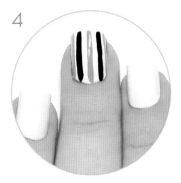

Clean the striping brush in acetone and load it with pink polish. Add pink stripes between the black stripes, allowing some of the base color to show through.

5

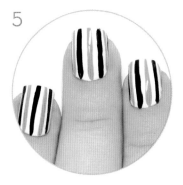

Follow steps 2 through 4 to create black and pink stripes on all of your nails. Allow to dry.

6

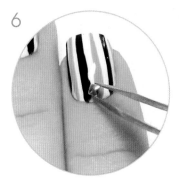

Apply a top coat to all nails. Using your nail art tweezers, place a nail stud in the wet top coat at the base of each nail.

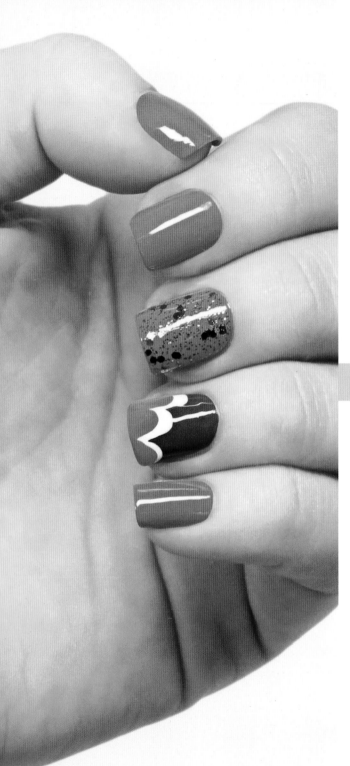

RUFFLE MANICURE

This abstract and graphic manicure design requires no special tools and works well with a variety of colors and finishes. The ruffle design also makes a great accent nail, as shown in this tutorial. Add a glitter nail to finish the look.

POLISH COLORS

Orange   Purple   White   Purple glitter

1

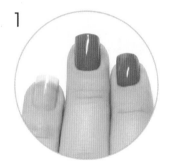

Polish all of your nails except for your ring finger with orange polish.

2

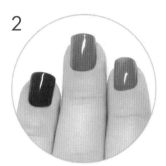

Polish your ring finger purple. This will be your ruffle accent nail.

3

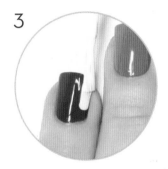

Apply one stroke of white polish near the sidewall of your ring finger nail, starting three-quarters of the way down your nail.

4

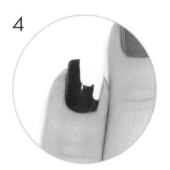

Repeat this technique in the center of your nail, starting about halfway down the nail and polishing to the free edge.

5

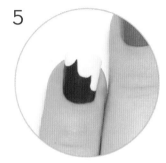

Repeat this technique again, near the other sidewall. Start from about one-quarter of the way down the nail and polish to the free edge.

6

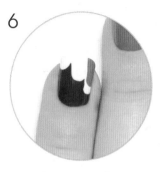

Using the same technique, apply an orange streak over the first white streak, allowing some white to show around the edges.

7

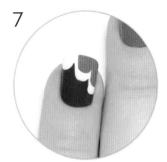

Apply the second orange streak near the middle of the nail. Again, allow some white to show.

8

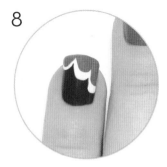

Apply a third orange streak, allowing white to show through at the bottom edge.

9

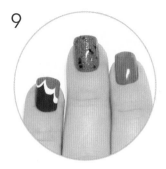

Polish your middle finger with a purple glitter polish, finishing your manicure.

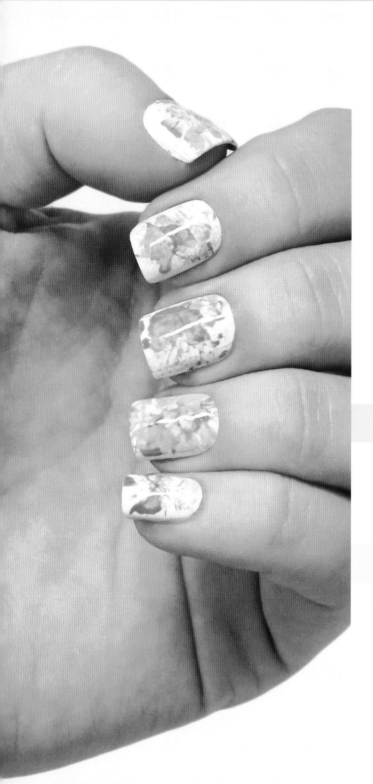

SPLATTER MANICURE

Everyone knows the best crafts are messy ones. To keep the mess to a minimum in this manicure, put pieces of tape around your nails to keep the polish off your skin. As always, you can clean up excess polish with acetone and an angled eyeliner brush.

MATERIALS

- Two straws
- Scissors
- Tape
- Polish palette
- Acetone
- Clean-up brush

POLISH COLORS

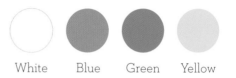

White   Blue   Green   Yellow

1

TAPE

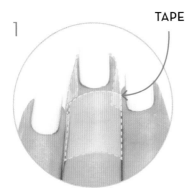

Cut drinking straws in half. Polish your nails white and carefully apply tape around your nails to aid in clean up.

2

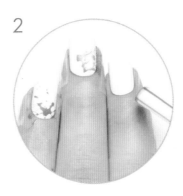

Dip a straw into a puddle of blue polish. Align the straw with your nail and blow through the clean end. Add blue splatters to all nails.

3

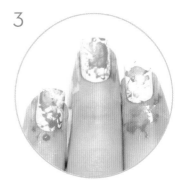

Dip a clean straw into green polish and repeat, adding green splatters to the nails.

4

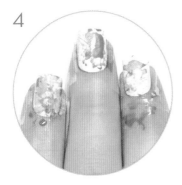

Repeat the splattering technique again with yellow polish.

5

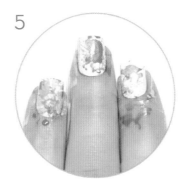

If needed, fill in empty space with splatters in any color.

6

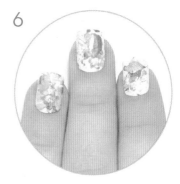

Remove tape and clean up with acetone and an angled eyeliner brush.

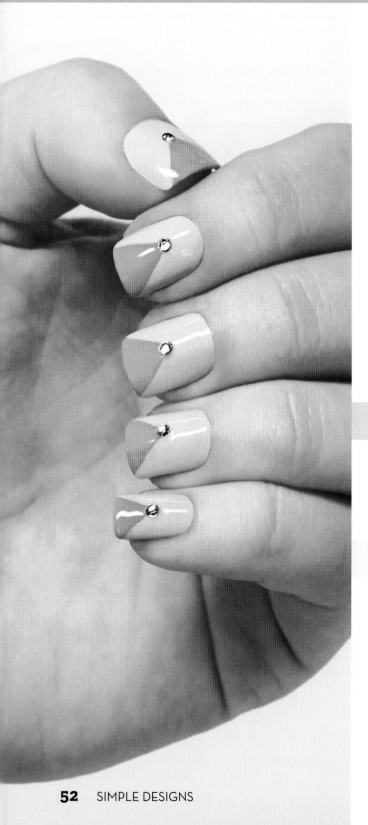

DEEP-V MANICURE

This fashion-forward twist on a French manicure is perfect for those who want a formal look without playing it too safe. Striping tape helps keep the lines crisp and clean, though you could do this freehand if you're confident in your brush skills.

MATERIALS

- Striping tape
- Striping brush
- Top coat
- Tweezers
- Rhinestones

POLISH COLORS

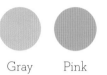

Gray   Pink

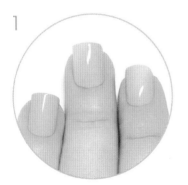

1

Polish your nails in gray polish. Let dry completely.

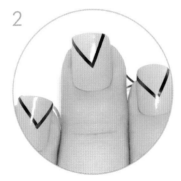

2

Apply two pieces of striping tape to each nail in a V-shape. Press onto nail.

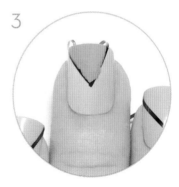

3

Polish the tip of one nail in pink polish, staying within the lines of the striping tape.

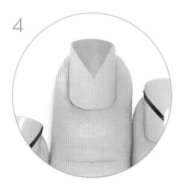

4

Remove the striping tape. Fix lines with your striping brush if there are any imperfections.

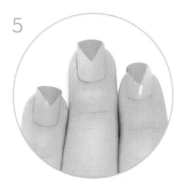

5

Repeat steps 3 and 4 on all of your nails, one nail at a time. Allow to dry completely.

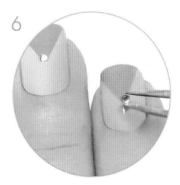

6

Apply a top coat to all nails. Use tweezers to set a rhinestone into the wet top coat at the apex of each deep-V.

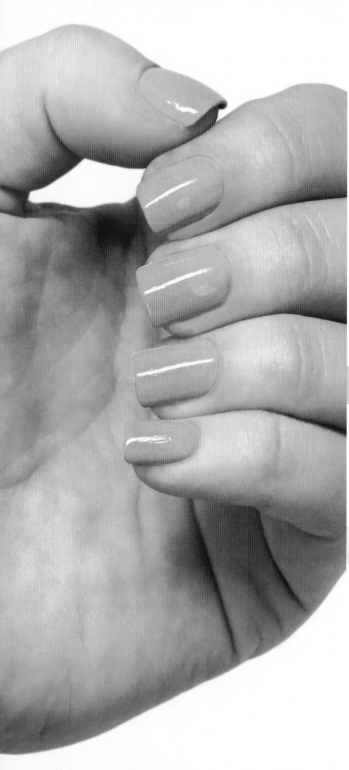

SIMPLE GRADIENT

One of the most popular nail art looks, the simple gradient can add something special to just about any manicure. Wear a gradient on its own or with nail art layered over the top for a special, textural manicure perfect for any occasion.

MATERIALS

- Cosmetic sponge
- Clean-up brush
- Acetone
- Top coat

POLISH COLORS

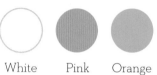

White   Pink   Orange

1

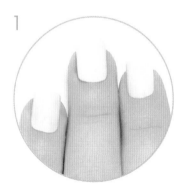

Polish your nails white and let dry.

2

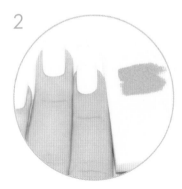

Paint side-by-side stripes of the gradient colors (in this case, pink and orange) onto a cosmetic sponge.

3

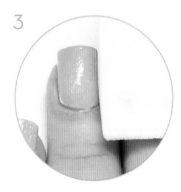

Stamp the polish onto your nails using gentle pressure.

4

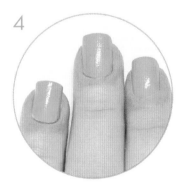

Repeatedly stamp the polish onto your nails, moving the sponge up and down slightly to blend the colors. Continue stamping until you achieve the gradient effect you desire.

5

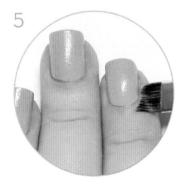

Use acetone and an angled eyeliner brush to remove excess polish from the skin.

6

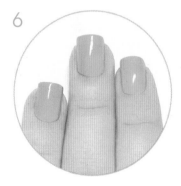

Apply a top coat to your nails to help blend the gradient and finish the look.

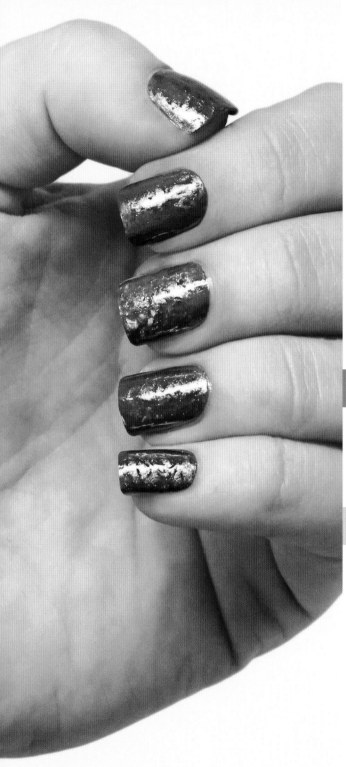

PLASTIC WRAP

Adding textural interest to your manicure can really step up the "wow" factor. Whether you wear this textured look on its own or as a base under beautiful nail art, you will be pleased with how simple it is to achieve.

MATERIALS

• Plastic wrap
• Acetone
• Clean-up brush

POLISH COLORS

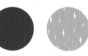

Blue   Gold

1

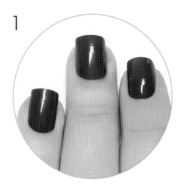

Polish your nails blue. Let dry.

2

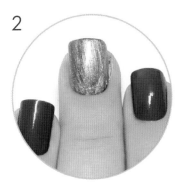

Paint a thick coat of gold polish over the dried blue polish on one nail.

3

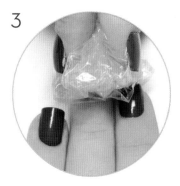

While the gold polish is still wet, stamp the nail with a scrunched-up piece of plastic wrap, lifting gold polish off the nail.

4

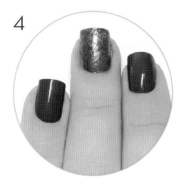

Apply more gold polish in sparse spots and "stamp" again until you achieve the textural effect you want.

5

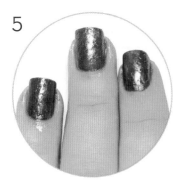

Repeat steps 2 through 4 on your other nails, one at a time.

6

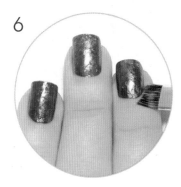

This technique will require clean up. Use acetone and an angled eyeliner brush.

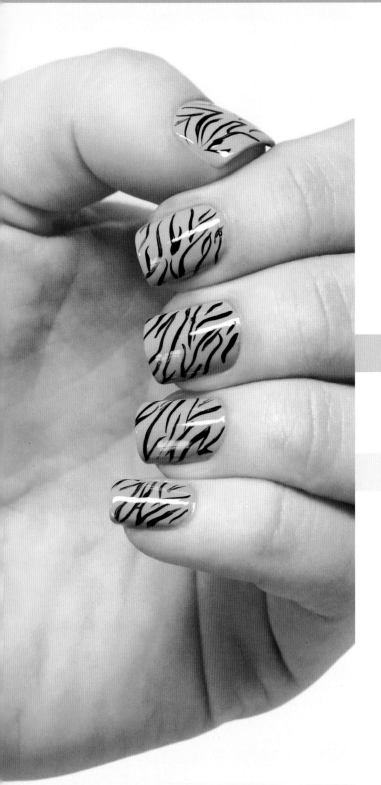

ZEBRA

Animal-print manicures can be girly and sassy, and zebra print is no exception. As you become comfortable with the basic method for creating zebra stripes, you will develop your own techniques for letting the stripes flow over the nail.

MATERIALS

- Striping brush
- Polish palette

POLISH COLORS

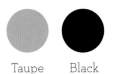

Taupe   Black

1

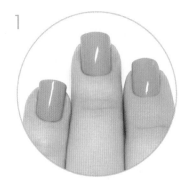

Polish your nails taupe.

2

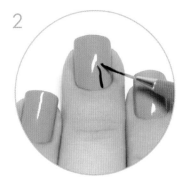

Load your striping brush with black polish or acrylic paint and create a V-shape at the corner of the nail.

3

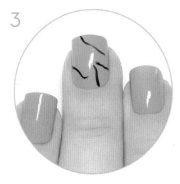

Paint two stripes coming in from the opposite side of the nail.

4

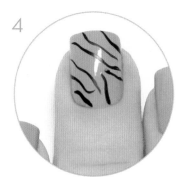

Between the stripes you just made, paint stripes coming from the same side of the nail as the original V-shape.

5

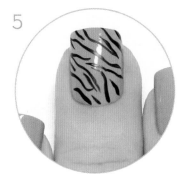

Add small lines to a few of the stripes, creating several more V-shapes and filling empty space on the nail.

6

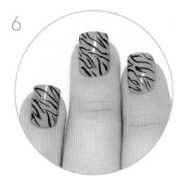

Finish your manicure by repeating steps 2 through 5 on all of your nails, or wear the zebra print as an accent nail.

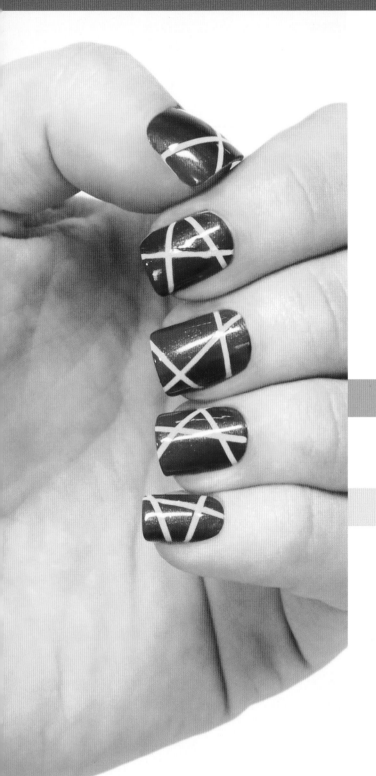

LASER MANICURE

Tape manicures require a lot of patience, but the finished look is always worth it. This manicure is graphic and eye-catching, and you can use a variety of contrasting color schemes to make your look really pop!

MATERIALS

• Striping tape

POLISH COLORS

Yellow   Pink

1

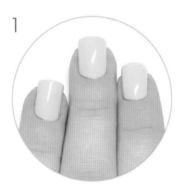

Polish your nails yellow. This will be the color of your laser beams. Let dry completely.

2

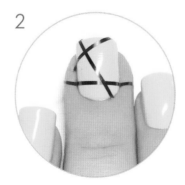

Apply three pieces of striping tape to each nail in an angular pattern.

3

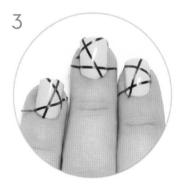

Rotate the orientation of the tape on each nail to create a more interesting finished manicure.

4

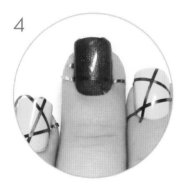

Apply pink polish over the striping tape on one nail.

5

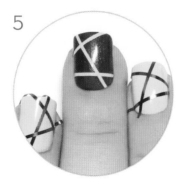

Immediately after polishing, carefully remove the striping tape, revealing your design.

6

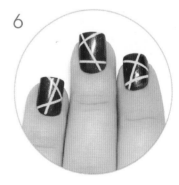

Repeat steps 4 and 5 on your remaining nails, finishing the manicure.

DRY BRUSH

Can't decide which polish to wear? Use this technique to combine them! This technique creates a textural finish that is perfect on its own or as a base under nail art. Use different polish colors and finishes to create a variety of looks with just the polish brush.

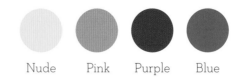

MATERIALS

• Paper towel

POLISH COLORS

Nude   Pink   Purple   Blue

1

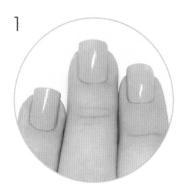

Polish your nails with nude polish. Allow to dry completely.

2

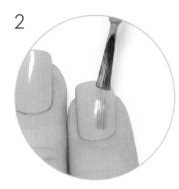

Remove the pink polish brush from the bottle and wipe nearly all the polish off on a paper towel. Gently drag the brush across the nail.

3

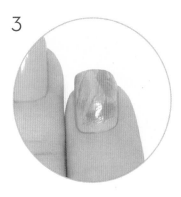

Repeat this all over the nail plate, at varying angles and lengths.

4

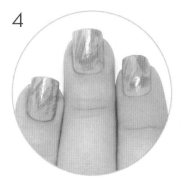

Repeat steps 2 and 3 to apply the pink dry brushing to all of your nails.

5

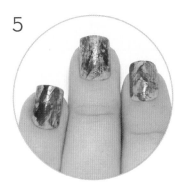

To create a more complex manicure, repeat steps 2 through 4 using a purple polish.

6

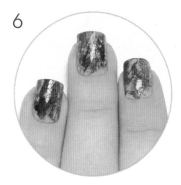

For an added layer of color, repeat steps 2 through 4 using a blue polish.

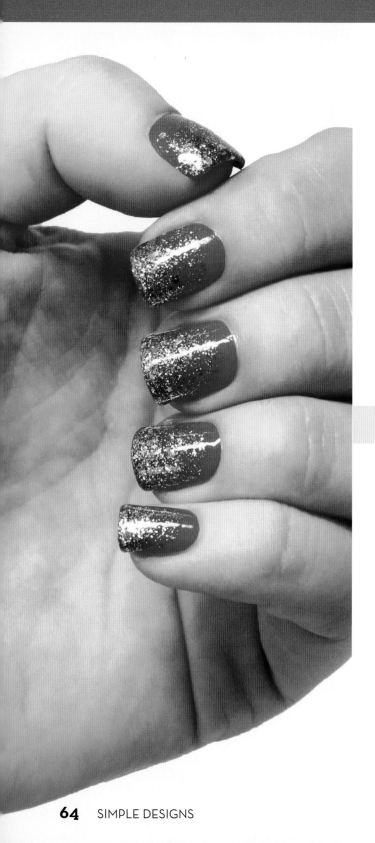

GLITTER GRADIENT

This modern, formal manicure will make you feel like a princess. You can use a cosmetic sponge to apply glitter to your tips, but this tutorial will teach you how to create a true gradient of sparkle using just the polish brush.

POLISH COLORS

Pink   Silver
              glitter

1

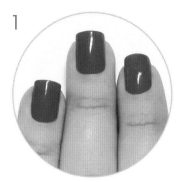

Polish your nails pink. Let dry.

2

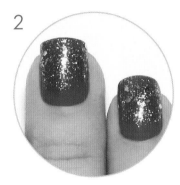

Using the brush from the bottle, apply a thin coat of silver glitter polish. Begin three-quarters down your nail and paint to the tip.

3

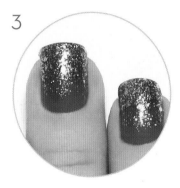

Using the same technique, apply another thin coat of silver glitter polish from half-way down the nail to the tip.

4

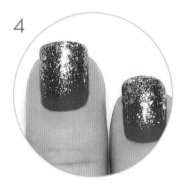

Apply a third thin coat of glitter, from one-quarter of the way down the nail to the tip. Don't let the polish get too thick on the nail.

5

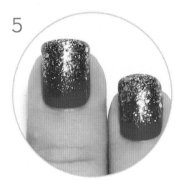

Add a final stroke of glitter polish right at the tip of the nail.

6

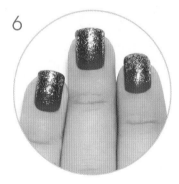

Fill in any space that is in need of glitter to make the gradient flow well.

SOUND WAVE MANICURE

The Sound Wave Manicure is a great way to bring together two of your favorite polish colors. Use this design as a simple, fun accent nail or wear it on all ten nails. Pink and gray are feminine and subtle, but you could also play with bold, contrasting colors.

MATERIALS

• Tape
• Striping brush
• Polish palette
• Top coat

POLISH COLORS

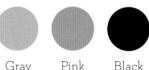

Gray   Pink   Black

1

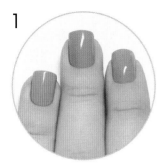

Polish your pinky and ring finger nails pink and your middle finger, pointer finger, and thumb nails gray. Let dry.

2

TAPE

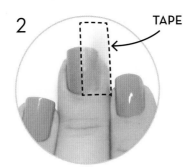

Apply a piece of tape to your middle finger nail, leaving the half nearest to your ring finger exposed.

3

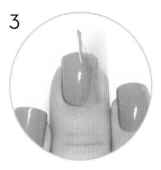

Polish the exposed part of your middle finger nail pink.

4

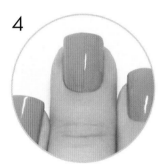

Immediately after polishing, remove the tape. If your line is not flawless, it's okay. This will be covered up.

5

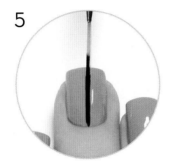

Using a striping brush and black polish or acrylic paint, paint a stripe down the center of the middle nail.

6

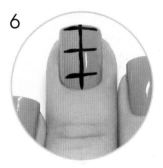

Paint three perpendicular lines along the length of the first vertical line.

7

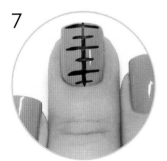

Paint three shorter perpendicular lines between each of the lines you created in step 6.

8

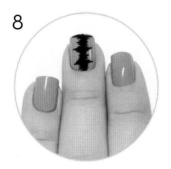

Begin painting more lines, creating a symmetric curve on each side of the sound wave.

9

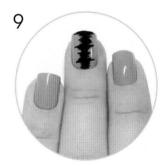

Fill in the curve with more lines so the sound wave is solid and nearly symmetrical. Finish with a top coat.

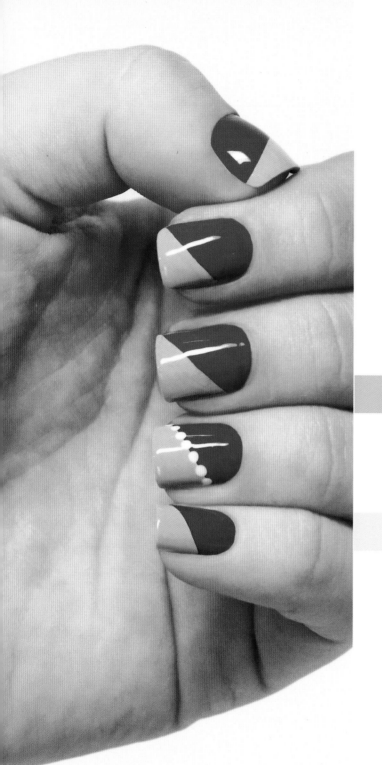

BASIC TAPE MANICURE

There are endless ways you can use tape to create straight lines in your manicures. This design uses tape to create an angled tip with polka-dot accents. Be creative and you'll be surprised how many designs you can come up with!

MATERIALS

• Tape
• Polish palette
• Dotting tool

POLISH COLORS

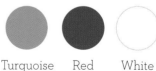

Turquoise   Red   White

1

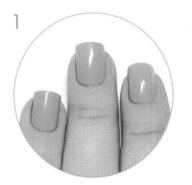

Polish your nails turquoise.
Let dry completely.

2

TAPE

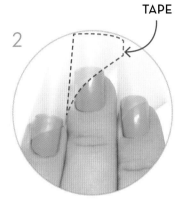

Apply a piece of stationery
tape to each nail at an angle,
covering the tip of the nail.

3

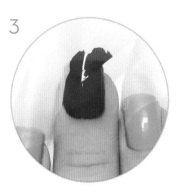

Polish the uncovered portion
of one nail with red polish.

4

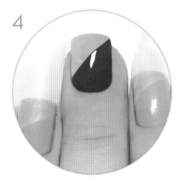

Immediately after applying
the red polish, remove the
tape. If the polish dries, your
lines won't be as crisp.

5

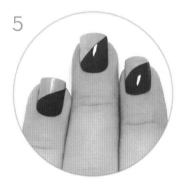

Repeat steps 3 and 4 on all of
your nails.

6

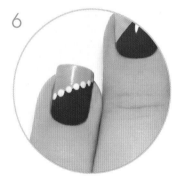

If desired, use your dotting
tool to add a few white polka
dots on your ring finger for a
fun accent nail.

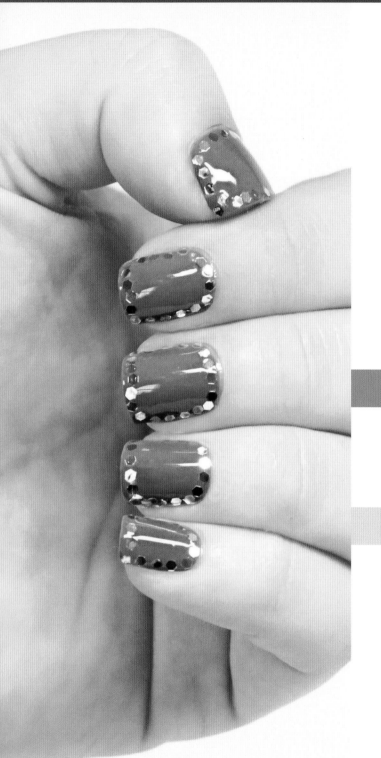

GLITTER FRAMES

You can use loose glitter to create striking sparkly accents. By carefully placing them around the edge of the nail, you will accentuate your nail shape and add just the perfect amount of bling to any manicure!

MATERIALS

- Top coat (not quick-dry)
- Dotting tool
- Loose glitter

POLISH COLORS

Purple

1

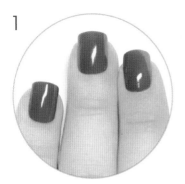

Polish your nails purple.
Let dry.

2

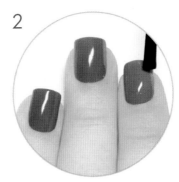

Apply top coat to one nail.

3

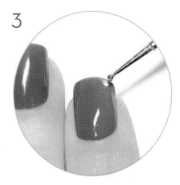

While the nail is wet, use a
dotting tool dipped in top
coat to pick up a piece of
glitter and apply it to your
nail, near the free edge.

4

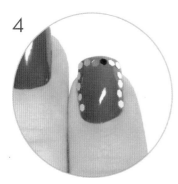

Continue placing glitter
pieces along the free edge
and down each sidewall.

5

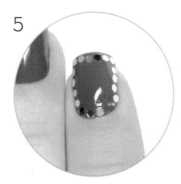

Finish by applying glitter
pieces along the curve at the
base of your nail.

6

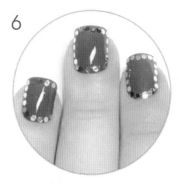

Repeat steps 2 through 5 to
place glitter on all nails. Seal
the glitter in with two layers of
top coat.

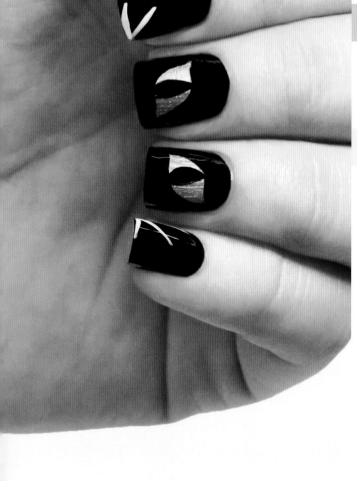

BLACK CAT

Halloween is the perfect time for a Black Cat manicure. This simple design is interesting because each nail is a bit different, but it comes together into a cohesive holiday look that is both spooky and adorable!

MATERIALS

• Striping brush
• Polish palette

POLISH COLORS

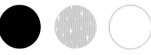

Black   Gold   White

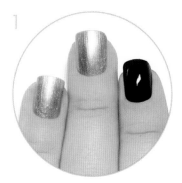

1

Polish your pointer and pinky nails black. Polish your remaining nails gold. Let dry for a few minutes.

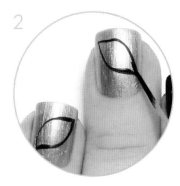

2

Using your striping brush and black polish or acrylic paint, create angled football-shaped eyes on the middle and ring finger nails.

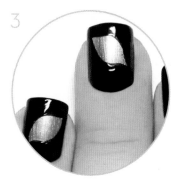

3

Use your striping brush to fill in the space around the eyes with black polish so that only the eye shapes are gold.

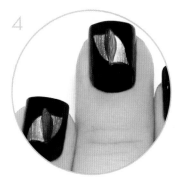

4

Using your striping brush and black polish or acrylic paint, create pupils in the eyes.

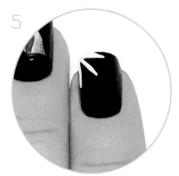

5

Using white polish or acrylic paint and your striping brush, create three lines coming from the corner of your pointer and pinky finger nails. These are the whiskers.

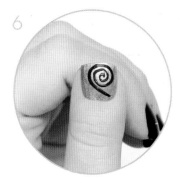

6

Using black polish or acrylic paint and your striping brush, carefully paint a swirl "tail" on your thumbnail.

SHINY-MATTE MANICURE

The Shiny-Matte Manicure is a great opportunity to play with contrasting polish finishes. This tutorial features a matte base and a shiny triangular design, but you can use shiny-matte contrast with many designs, such as dots, zebra, and leopard.

MATERIALS

- Matte top coat
- Top coat
- Striping brush
- Polish palette

POLISH COLORS

Black

1

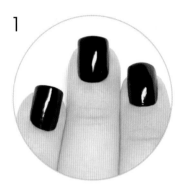

Polish your nails black.

2

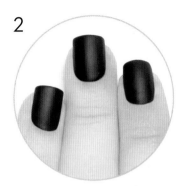

Apply matte top coat to all of your nails. Let dry.

3

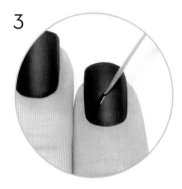

Using your striping brush and clear top coat, paint a line from the corner to the center of your nail plate.

4

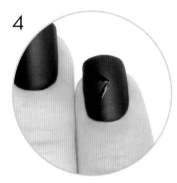

Repeat step 3 from the free edge to the center.

5

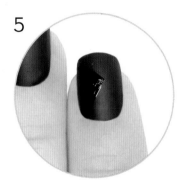

Fill in the triangle with clear top coat using your striping brush.

6

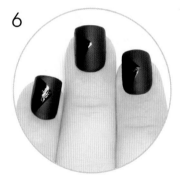

Complete steps 3 through 5 on all of your nails for a monochromatic, trendy look.

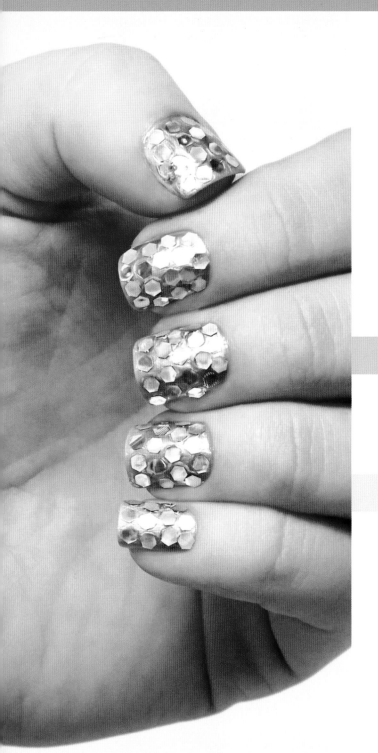

DISCO BALL

When you have a special occasion and your nails need to look the part, it doesn't get any more special than the Disco Ball nail. This design is simple to do, and the sparkle payoff is huge! Wear this as a full manicure or a fun accent nail.

MATERIALS

- Top coat (not quick-dry)
- Dotting tool
- Loose silver glitter

POLISH COLORS

Silver

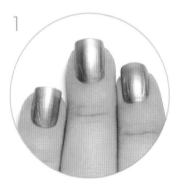

1

Polish your nails silver.
Let dry.

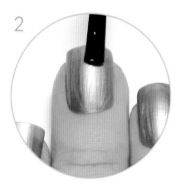

2

Apply a coat of top coat to
one nail.

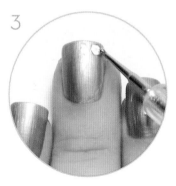

3

Use a dotting tool dipped in
top coat to pick up a silver
glitter piece and place it on
your nail.

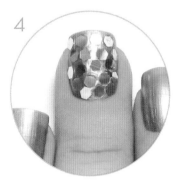

4

Continue placing glitter
pieces on your nail until
the nail plate is completely
covered in glitter.

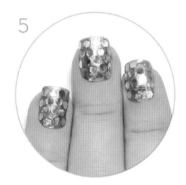

5

Repeat steps 2 through 4 on
all of your nails, completing
one nail at a time.

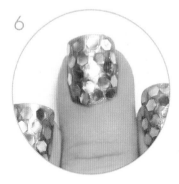

6

Seal in the glitter with two
coats of top coat.

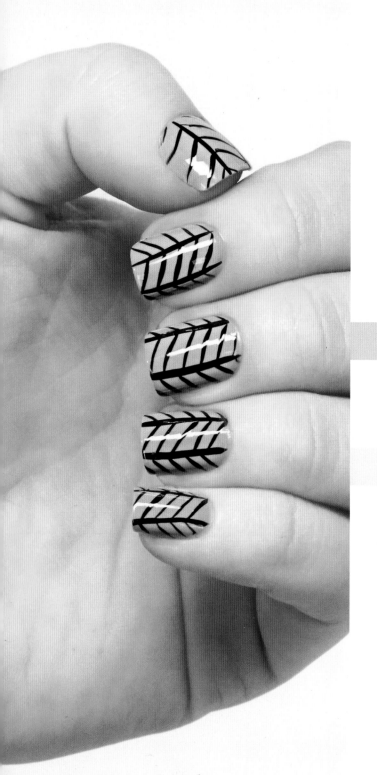

HERRINGBONE

Sometimes less is more. Using just straight lines, you can create a fun herringbone design that looks great over any polish color or finish. You can keep it classic over a neutral base or play it up with a brighter color, as shown here.

MATERIALS

• Striping brush
• Polish palette

POLISH COLORS

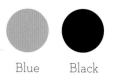

Blue   Black

1

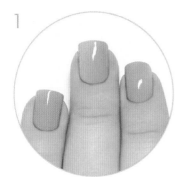

Polish your nails blue. Let dry for a few minutes.

2

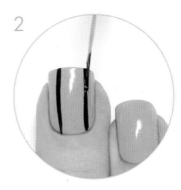

Using your striping brush and black polish or acrylic paint, paint two vertical stripes on your nail.

3

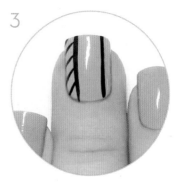

Using the striping brush and black polish or acrylic paint, create short lines angling up from the sidewall to the first vertical stripe.

4

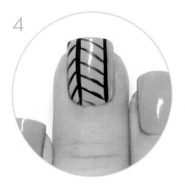

Paint short lines angling down between the two vertical lines.

5

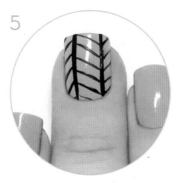

Paint a final set of short lines, this time angled-up, between the second vertical line and other sidewall.

6

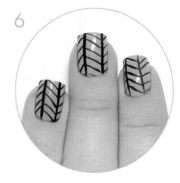

Finish your manicure by repeating steps 2 through 5 on all of your nails.

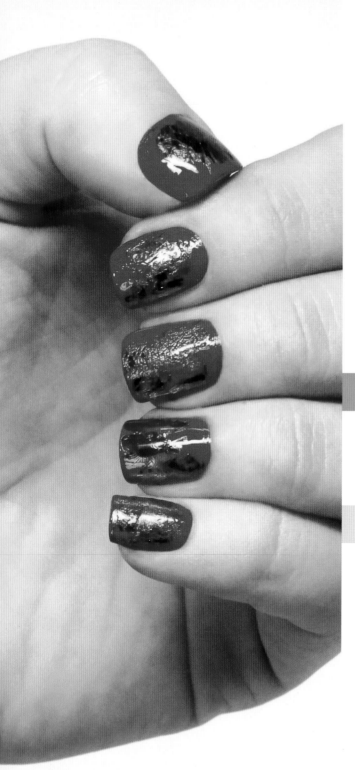

FOIL ACCENTS

Nail foils can add a glitzy glow to any classic manicure. This technique requires no special tools aside from the nail foils, which are available in countless colors and designs. Here, red foil and red polish create a glowing monochromatic look.

MATERIALS

- Scissors
- Red nail foils
- Top coat

POLISH COLORS

Red

1

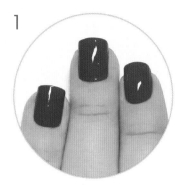

Polish your nails red. Let dry until just tacky.

2

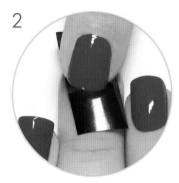

Cut a piece of nail foil to approximately fit your nail and gently press it onto your tacky nail.

3

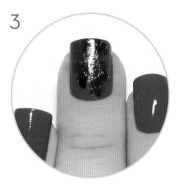

Carefully lift the foil off the nail, leaving some of the shiny foil behind. This technique creates a textured, marbled look.

4

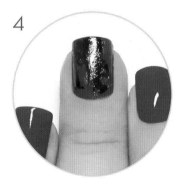

Repeat this process until you are pleased with the effect on your nail.

5

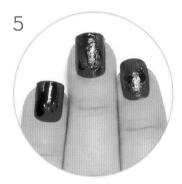

Repeat steps 2 through 4 on each nail. If the polish dries, apply top coat and let dry until tacky and proceed.

6

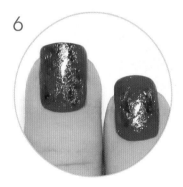

Seal in nail foil with two layers of top coat.

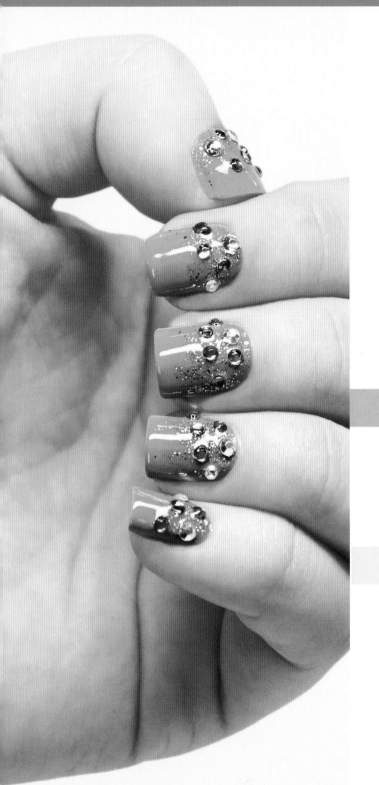

RHINESTONE ACCENTS

Nothing is flashier than rhinestones and crystals, especially on your nails. By using a variety of rhinestones in different colors, sizes, and shapes, you can create a texturally interesting manicure that looks complex but requires little effort.

MATERIALS

- Top coat (not quick-dry)
- Nail glue
- Tweezers
- Rhinestones

POLISH COLORS

Blue   Silver glitter

1

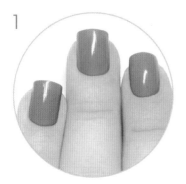

Polish your nails blue. Let dry.

2

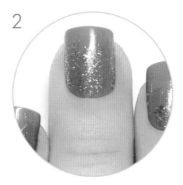

Polish each nail with a splash of silver glitter polish, starting from the cuticle to about halfway up the nail.

3

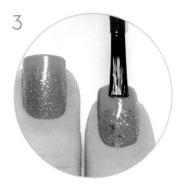

Apply a coat of top coat to one nail. For longer-lasting stones, use nail glue instead.

4

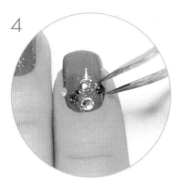

While the top coat or glue is wet, use tweezers to apply a variety of rhinestones over the glitter polish.

5

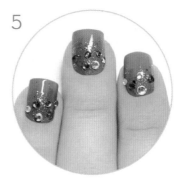

Repeat steps 3 and 4 on your other nails. Add stones until you are happy with the effect.

6

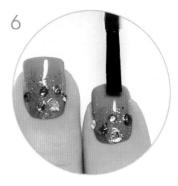

Once dry, carefully apply a thick coat of top coat over the stones.

RHINESTONE ACCENTS   **83**

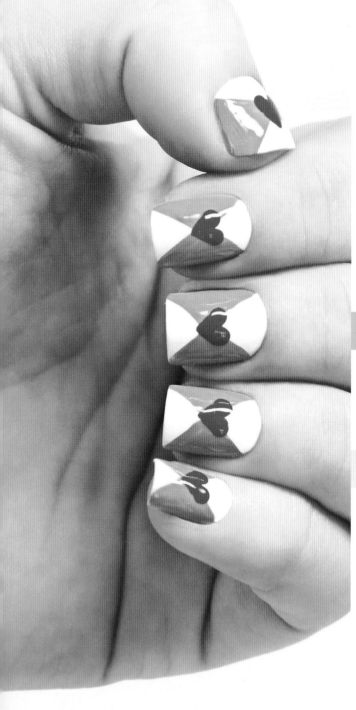

FLOATING HEART

Hearts can be created using a dotting tool and striping brush. With practice, hearts will become a crucial part of your nail art skill set. In this manicure, romantic colors come together for a perfect Valentine's Day look.

MATERIALS

• Striping brush
• Dotting tool
• Polish palette

POLISH COLORS

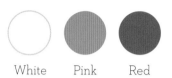

White   Pink   Red

1

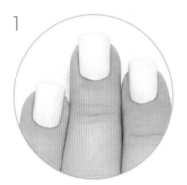

Polish your nails white. Let dry for a few minutes.

2

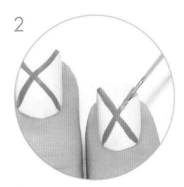

Using your striping brush, paint a pink "X" on each nail.

3

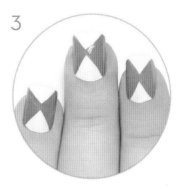

Using your striping brush, fill in the sides of the "X" with pink polish. Let dry briefly.

4

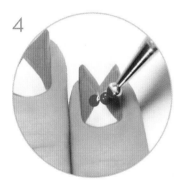

To create the heart, make two red dots close together in the center of one nail.

5

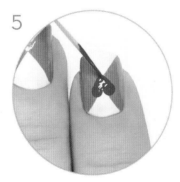

Use your striping brush loaded with red polish to gently pull the dots down to a point to create a heart.

6

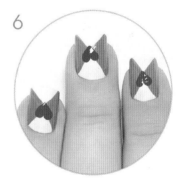

Complete steps 4 and 5 on each nail.

CHECKER-BOARDS

Bold black-and-white checkerboard nails are perfect for a punk rock show or a weekend at the racetrack. Pair a checkerboard accent nail with a bright neon manicure for a fun, contrasting look.

MATERIALS

- Striping brush
- Polish palette
- Top coat

POLISH COLORS

White   Black

1

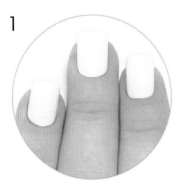

Polish your nails white.

2

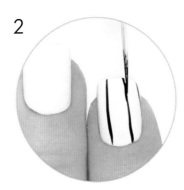

Using your striping brush and black polish or acrylic paint, create two or three evenly spaced vertical lines on your nail.

3

In a similar fashion, create horizontal lines, making a grid of squares on the nail.

4

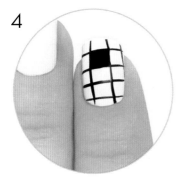

Using the tip of your striping brush, fill in one square in the grid.

5

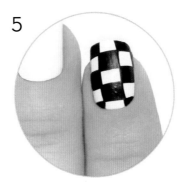

Continue out from the black square, filling in the grid in a staggered pattern.

6

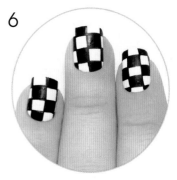

Complete steps 2 through 5 on the rest of your nails, or wear the checkerboard design as an accent nail. Add a top coat to complete the look.

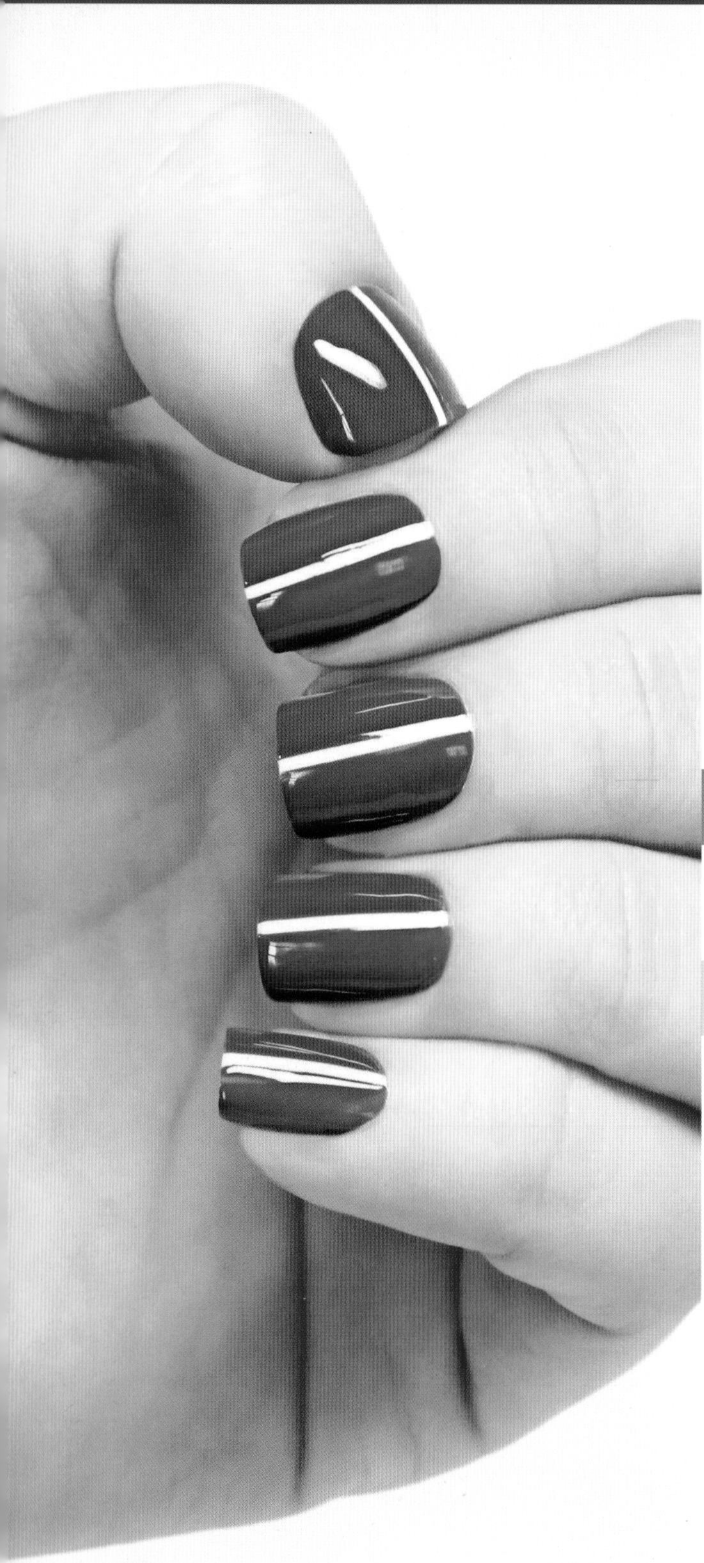

VERTICAL LINE

This striping tape design allows you to use several of your favorite polish shades in one manicure. Choose bold, contrasting shades for a wild look or multiple polishes from the same color family for a more subtle manicure.

MATERIALS

• Striping tape

POLISH COLORS

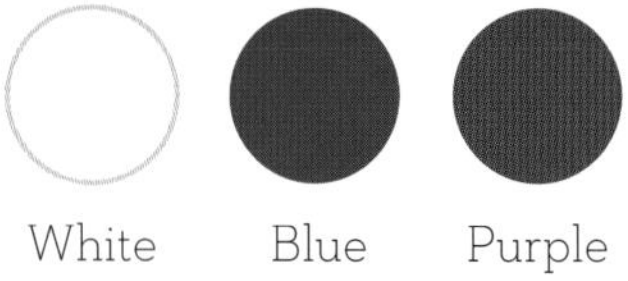

White   Blue   Purple

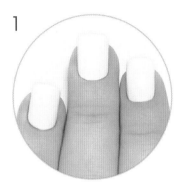

1

Polish your nails white. Let dry completely.

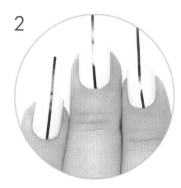

2

Apply a single piece of striping tape down the center of each nail.

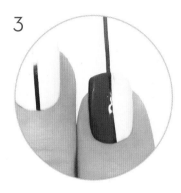

3

Polish half of one nail blue, being careful not to cross over the striping tape.

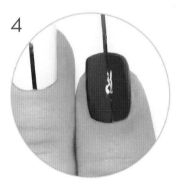

4

Polish the other half of the nail purple, again being careful not to paint over the tape.

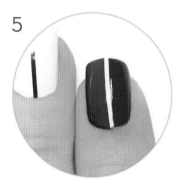

5

Immediately after polishing, remove the striping tape. If the polish dries before you remove it, the line will not be as crisp.

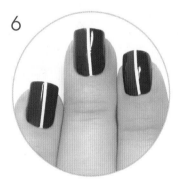

6

Repeat steps 3 through 5 on the rest of your nails.

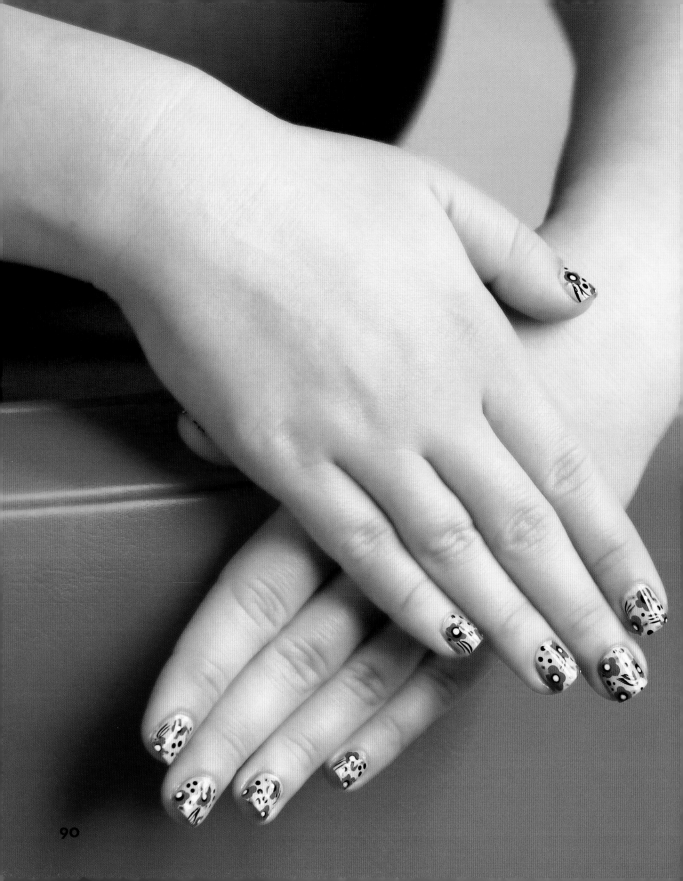

INTERMEDIATE DESIGNS

The intermediate nail art designs in this section require more freehand work, but once you have mastered a few simple strokes with your striping brush, you will find them well within your skill set. Between graphic patterns and holiday-themed manicures, you will find something perfect for any occasion. The tutorials can be adapted to work with many color schemes and polish finishes, so be creative and design something that is truly you!

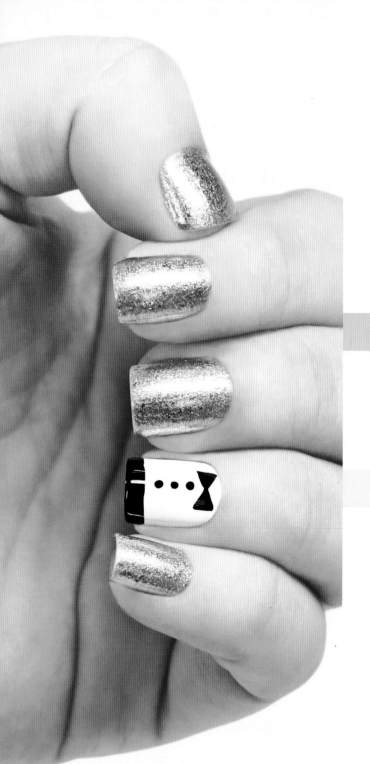

TUXEDO NAIL

When you attend a formal affair, your nails need to look the part as well. Adorn your nails in their own black tie and you will have a conversation starter worthy of the runway at your fingertips.

MATERIALS

• Tape
• Striping brush
• Dotting tool
• Polish palette

POLISH COLORS

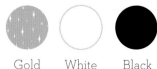

Gold   White   Black

1

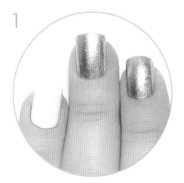

Polish your nails gold with a white accent nail.

2

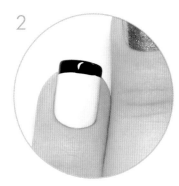

Paint a black French tip on the white nail. Use tape for this if it's easier for you.

3

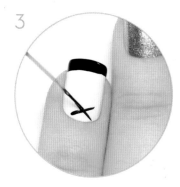

Near the base of your nail, paint an "X" shape in black polish or acrylic paint with your striping brush.

4

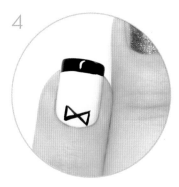

Paint two small lines to close off the "X" into a bowtie shape.

5

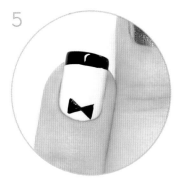

Using your striping brush, carefully fill in the bowtie.

6

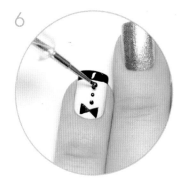

Using black polish and your dotting tool, create two or three "buttons" down the center of the nail.

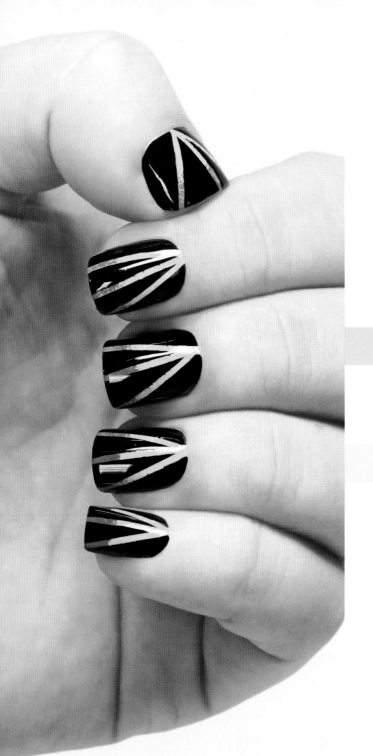

SUNBURST

By combining sponging and striping tape techniques, you can create a wide variety of bold, graphic looks. In this manicure, the tape is lifted to reveal a gradation of summertime colors that really pop against the black polish.

MATERIALS

• Cosmetic sponge
• Striping tape

POLISH COLORS

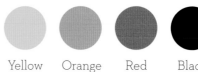

Yellow   Orange   Red   Black

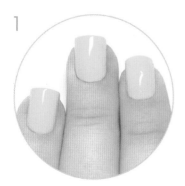

1

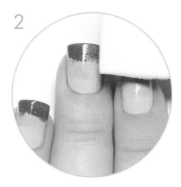

2

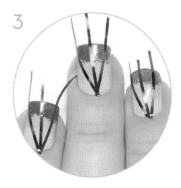

3

Polish your nails yellow. Let dry completely.

Use a cosmetic sponge to apply orange polish to the half of your nail closest to the free edge and red polish to the tip of each nail. Let dry.

Apply three pieces of striping tape to each nail, in a fan shape, starting at the cuticle.

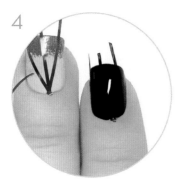

4

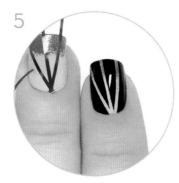

5

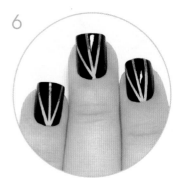

6

Polish over the striping tape with black polish on one nail.

Immediately after polishing (before it dries), carefully remove the striping tape to reveal the color underneath.

Repeat steps 4 and 5 on the rest of your nails.

TREE NAIL

Whatever the season, trees are always a whimsical motif to use in nail art. This tutorial shows you how to create a basic tree, but as you become more comfortable with your striping brush, you can create larger, more flowing trees.

MATERIALS

• Striping brush
• Polish palette

POLISH COLORS

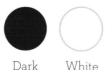

Dark green   White

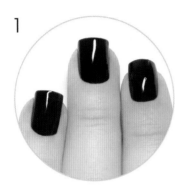

1

Polish your nails dark green.

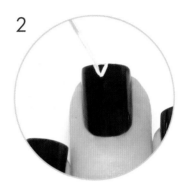

2

Using white polish or acrylic paint and your striping brush, paint a small triangle at the tip of your nail.

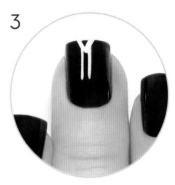

3

Paint two vertical lines coming down from the small triangle, creating the "trunk" of the tree.

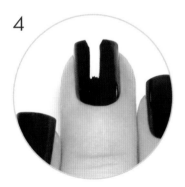

4

Use your striping brush to fill in the tree trunk.

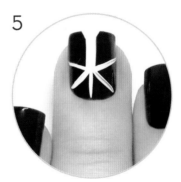

5

Paint several thick lines coming out of the trunk. These are the main branches.

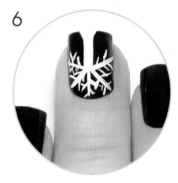

6

Paint several thinner, shorter lines off of each thicker branch, completing the tree.

GLITTER HEART

Heart manicures are classic for Valentine's Day or any time you want to celebrate love. This manicure combines soft, feminine shades with sparkling glitter, a contrast that is always in style.

MATERIALS

- Top coat (not quick-dry)
- Dotting tool
- Pink hexagonal glitter

POLISH COLORS

Gray   Pink

1

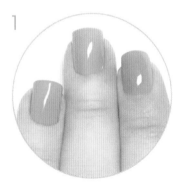

Paint your nails gray with a pink accent nail on your ring finger. Let dry.

2

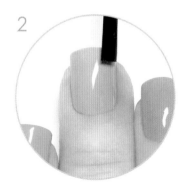

On your middle finger, apply a coat of top coat.

3

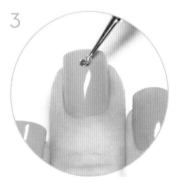

Using a dotting tool dipped in top coat, place a pink glitter piece onto your nail, centered near the free edge.

4

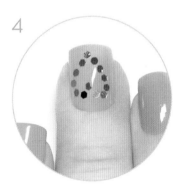

Continue placing glitter pieces on your nail, creating the outline of a heart.

5

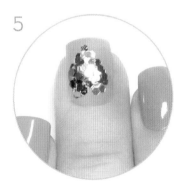

Continue using glitter pieces to fill in the heart shape.

6

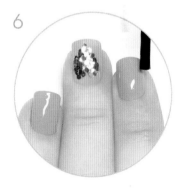

Seal in the glitter with two coats of top coat.

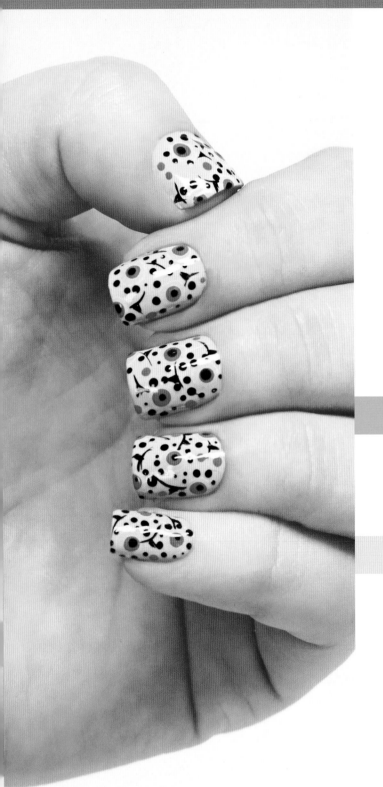

BOHO FLORAL

This funky floral pattern requires nothing more than dots and a few simple strokes with your striping brush. Once it's complete, you'll be ready for the beach or a summer festival. Combine bold, contrasting shades for an eye-catching look.

MATERIALS

• Dotting tool
• Polish palette
• Striping brush

POLISH COLORS

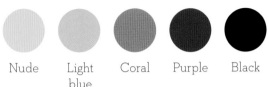

| Nude | Light blue | Coral | Purple | Black |

1

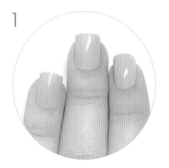

Paint your nails in a nude polish. Let dry for a few minutes.

2

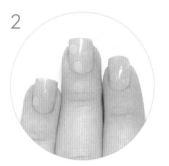

Use your dotting tool to create large light blue dots evenly spaced across your nails.

3

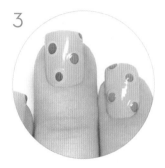

Clean your dotting tool and then use it to place a dot of coral polish in the center of each blue dot.

4

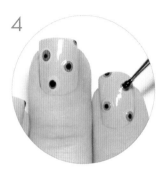

Use the smaller end of your dotting tool to place small purple dots in the center of each coral dot. These are your flowers.

5

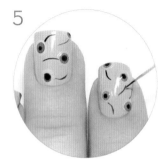

Using your striping brush and black polish or acrylic paint, paint small, curved lines from each flower.

6

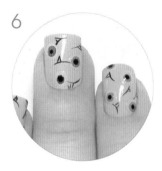

Using your striping brush again, paint a small triangle "leaf" coming from each stem.

7

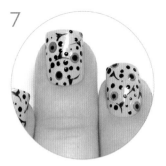

Carefully fill in each triangle-shaped leaf with black polish or acrylic paint.

8

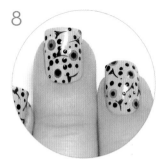

Using your dotting tool and black polish, place small black dots around each flower shape. They may overlap each other.

9

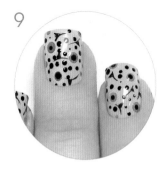

Fill in any empty space on the nail with coral dots.

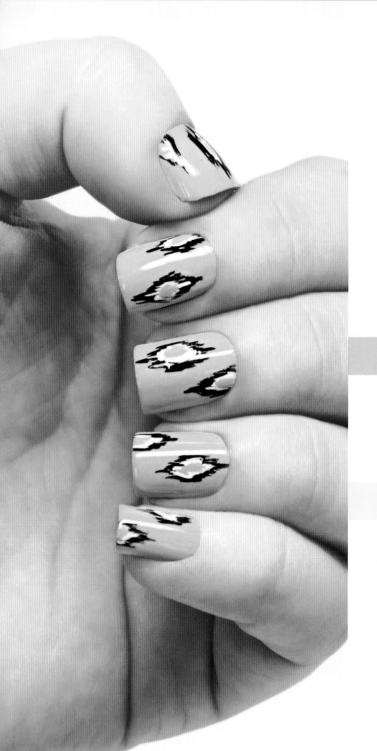

IKAT

Graphic-patterned nails work well for most occasions and all ages. This design, inspired by ikat textile patterns, is easy to create because none of the lines are precise. You can use any polish colors you'd like to match your outfit or mood.

MATERIALS

- Striping brush
- Polish palette
- Top coat

POLISH COLORS

Blue   Black   White

1

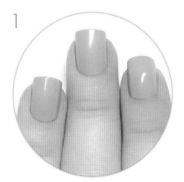

Polish your nails blue. Let dry for a few minutes.

2

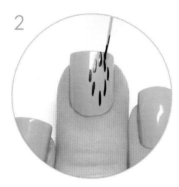

Using a striping brush and black polish or acrylic paint, paint a series of short, black, vertical lines on one nail, outlining a diamond shape.

3

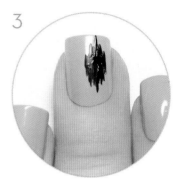

Fill the outline in with more vertical black lines, creating a more solid diamond shape.

4

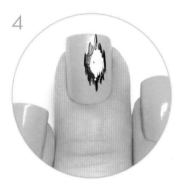

Using white polish or acrylic paint and your striping brush, paint a similar smaller white diamond shape within the black one.

5

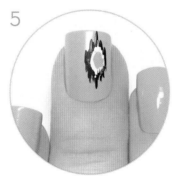

Use your striping brush to add a small blue diamond in the center of the white diamond.

6

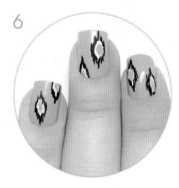

Repeat steps 2 through 5, spacing out the pattern across all of your nails. Add a top coat to complete the look.

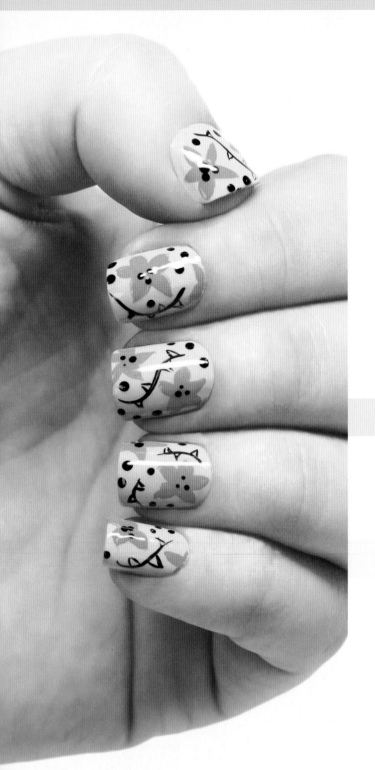

TROPICAL FLORAL

Tropical flowers are perfect for vacation manicures and pedicures. This tutorial shows how to create an all-over floral print, but you could easily paint just one flower at the base of each nail (or toenail) for a chic look.

MATERIALS

• Striping brush
• Polish palette
• Dotting tool

POLISH COLORS

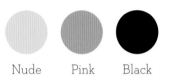

Nude   Pink   Black

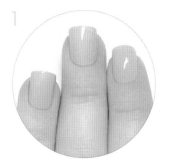

1

Polish your nails a nude shade.

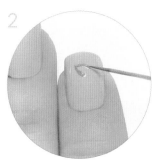

2

Using your striping brush loaded with pink polish, paint two curved brushstrokes that meet at a point.

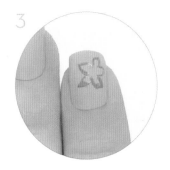

3

Repeat step 2, creating a flower shape with five petals. You can also make four-point flowers.

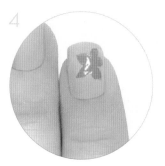

4

Use your striping brush to fill in the flower shape with pink polish.

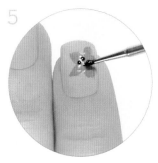

5

Using your dotting tool and black polish, create three small dots in the center of the flower.

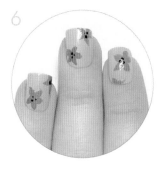

6

Repeat steps 2 through 5, filling your nails with flowers. For a complete look, create some partial flowers at the edges of your nails.

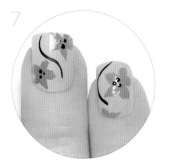

7

Use your striping brush loaded with black polish or acrylic paint to create curved lines between the flowers.

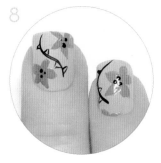

8

Use your striping brush to carefully add triangle-shaped leaves to the lines.

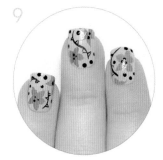

9

Using your dotting tool and black polish, fill any empty space on your nails with small dots.

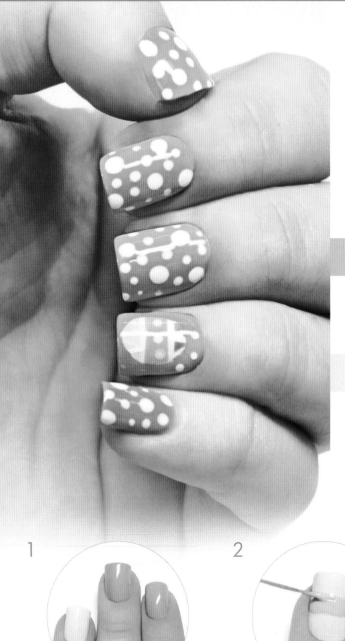

EASTER EGG

In the springtime, pastel egg motifs are all around. This cute, patterned design makes a great accent nail paired with multi-sized polka dots.

MATERIALS

- Striping brush
- Polish palette
- Dotting tool
- Top coat

POLISH COLORS

Pastel yellow   Pastel pink   Pastel purple   Orange   White

1

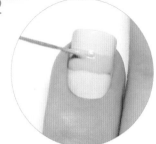

Polish your nails orange with a pastel yellow accent nail. The pastel nail will be your Easter egg nail.

2

On your accent nail, use your striping brush and pastel pink polish to create a horizontal stripe in the center of your nail.

3

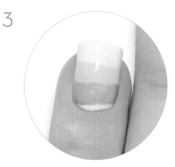

Using a similar method, paint a pastel purple horizontal stripe below the pink one you just created.

4

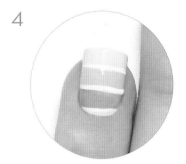

Using your striping brush loaded with white polish or acrylic paint, make straight lines above and below the pastel stripes where they meet.

5

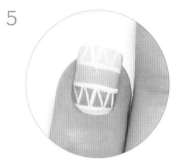

Use your striping brush and white polish or acrylic paint to create tiny zigzags on the yellow and purple stripes.

6

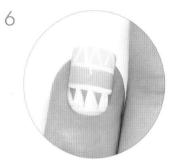

Carefully fill in the staggered triangles you just created within the zigzags on the purple stripe.

7

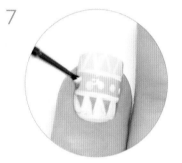

Use your dotting tool and white polish to create small dots on the pink stripe.

8

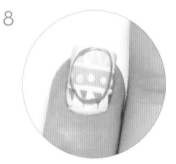

Use your striping brush and orange polish to carefully outline the shape of an egg over the pastel design you just created.

9

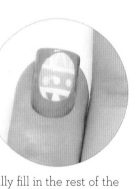

Carefully fill in the rest of the nail with orange polish, revealing an egg shape filled with pretty designs.

10

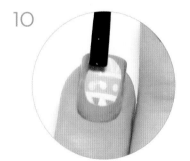

Paint the accent nail with a top coat to smooth out the patterned design.

11

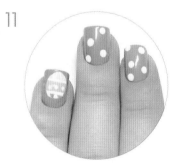

Use your dotting tool and white polish to create several large dots, spaced randomly across your orange-polished nails.

12

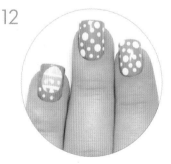

Fill in the space left on the nails using the small end of your dotting tool and white polish.

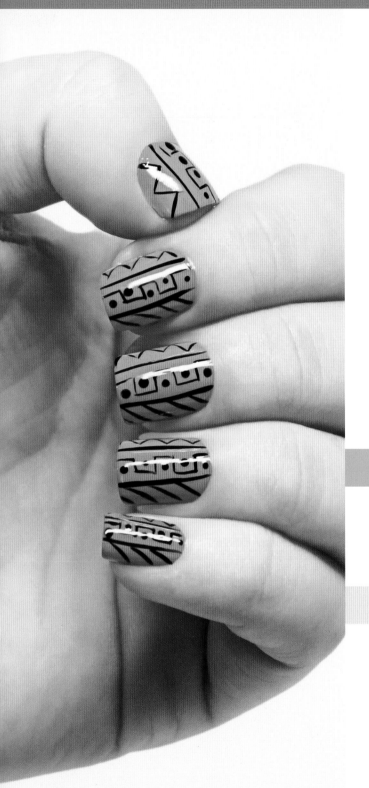

GEOMETRIC MANICURE

Geometric manicures are graphic and trendy. This tutorial outlines several patterns that work well together, but be creative! You can make countless designs using nothing more than straight lines and dots. Pair a geometric print with a textural or gradient background for an impressive manicure.

MATERIALS

• Striping brush
• Polish palette
• Dotting tool

POLISH COLORS

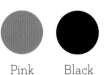

Pink   Black

1

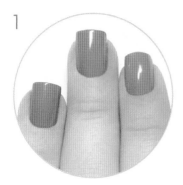

Polish your nails pink.

2

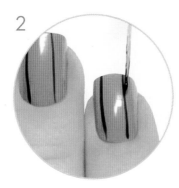

Using your striping brush and black polish or acrylic paint, create two vertical lines on each nail.

3

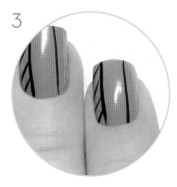

Using your striping brush again, paint short upward-slanting lines between the sidewall and the first vertical line.

4

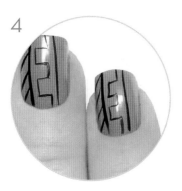

Between the two vertical lines, carefully paint small line segments, creating the geometric pattern shown.

5

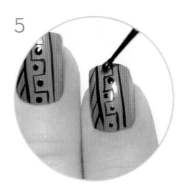

Using your dotting tool and black polish, place a small dot in each notch of the design you just made.

6

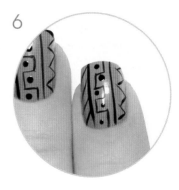

Using your striping brush, create a zigzag line between the second vertical line and the sidewall.

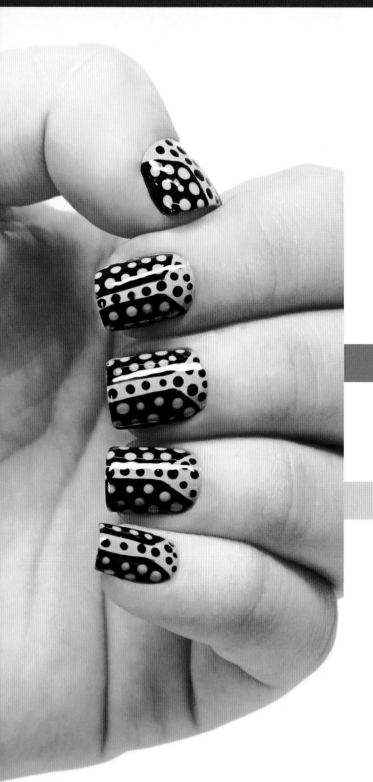

V-GAPS

Can't decide which of your two favorite polishes to wear? Use them both in this fun design. Simple lines and dots in contrasting colors virtually pop off the nail. For a subtler look, skip the polka dots or use polishes of the same hue.

MATERIALS

- Striping brush
- Polish palette
- Dotting tool

POLISH COLORS

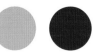

Gray   Dark
              purple

1

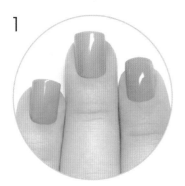

Polish your nails gray. Let dry for a few minutes.

2

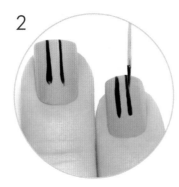

Using your striping brush and dark purple polish, paint two vertical lines from the tip of your nail that stop about two-thirds of the way down.

3

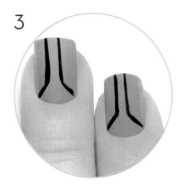

Paint two more lines at an angle from the first ones, connecting to the corner of your nail near the cuticle.

4

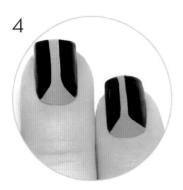

Carefully fill in the shapes you just created near the sidewalls, leaving the gray center exposed.

5

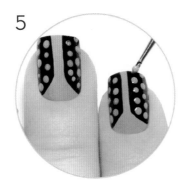

Using your dotting tool, fill the dark purple areas with small gray dots.

6

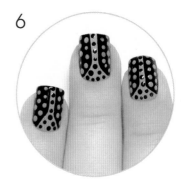

Again using your dotting tool, fill the gray area with small, dark purple dots.

SPLASH FLORAL

Bright and springy, the Splash Floral manicure is perfect for warm weather or those who want to start with subtle nail art. This manicure uses a bright yellow color scheme, but pink, purple, or lime green would work wonderfully as well.

MATERIALS

- Striping brush
- Polish palette
- Dotting tool

POLISH COLORS

Yellow   White   Black

1

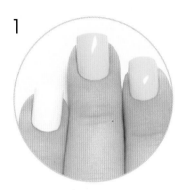

Polish your nails yellow with a white accent nail. Let dry for a few minutes.

2

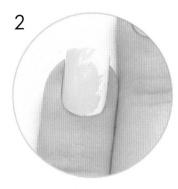

Remove the brush from the yellow polish bottle and wipe off most of the polish. On the white nail, use the dry brush to create a splash of color coming up from the cuticle.

3

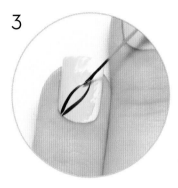

Using your striping brush and black polish or acrylic paint, create a petal shape over the yellow splash. Flowing strokes work best.

4

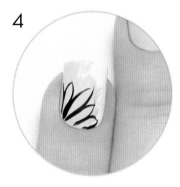

Create several more petals, filling the corner of your nail.

5

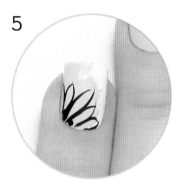

Using your dotting tool and black polish, create two or three small dots in the center of the flower.

6

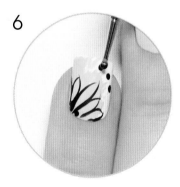

To create some movement on the nail, add three small dots in a curved shape toward the tip of the nail.

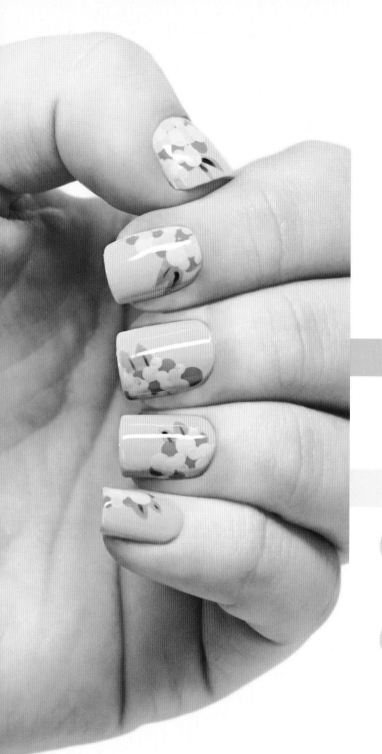

HYDRANGEAS

Few flowers are more stylish or romantic than blue hydrangeas. This technique combines several shades of blue to create the iconic blooms using simple polka dots. When paired with a soft pink, this manicure is perfect for a springtime wedding.

MATERIALS

• Dotting tool
• Polish palette
• Striping brush

POLISH COLORS

  Light green

Soft pink   True blue   Light green   Dark green

Light blue   Medium blue

1

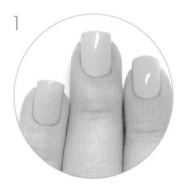

Polish your nails soft pink.

2

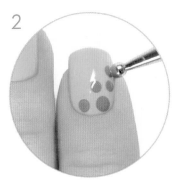

On each nail, create a cluster of true blue dots. You can place them in different spots on each nail.

3

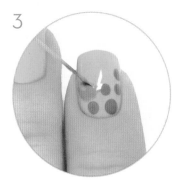

Using your striping brush and a light green polish, paint two triangular leaves coming off each cluster of blue dots.

4

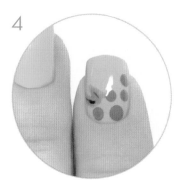

Using your striping brush and dark green polish, add an accent line down the center of each leaf.

5

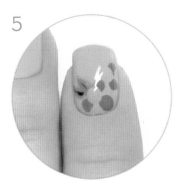

Add light blue dots to the cluster you started in step 2, covering the edges of the leaves.

6

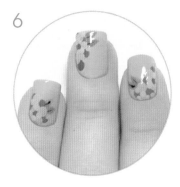

Complete the flowers with more dots in a medium blue shade, being sure to cover most of the pink polish.

POPPY FLORAL

This all-over floral pattern features autumnal colors, but you could wear this design any time of year. Whimsical details and dots in this manicure make it original and eye-catching.

MATERIALS

- Dotting tool
- Polish palette
- Striping brush

POLISH COLORS

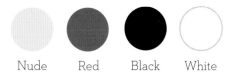

Nude   Red   Black   White

Light green   Dark green   Brown

1

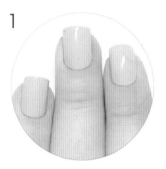

Polish your nails in a nude shade.

2

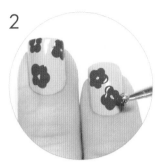

Use your dotting tool and red polish to create five dots connected in a circular fashion. Space them over your nails.

3

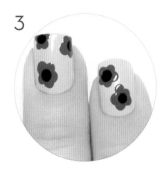

Use your dotting tool and black polish to add a black dot in the center of each flower.

4

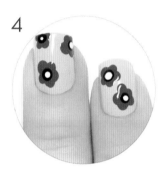

Use the small end of your dotting tool and white polish to add a small white dot to the center of each flower.

5

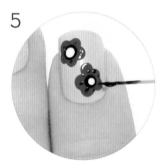

Using the tip of your striping brush and black polish, add tiny dots around the black center of each flower.

6

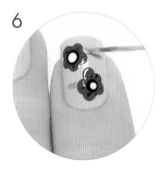

Use your striping brush and a light green polish to create triangular leaves coming off each flower.

7

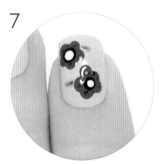

Use your striping brush and a dark green polish to add an accent line down the center of each leaf.

8

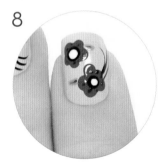

Using your striping brush and black polish, create short, curved lines coming from a few of the flowers.

9

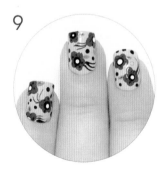

Fill any empty space on your nails with small, brown dots.

SPIDERWEBS

Halloween is the perfect time to dress up your fingertips! Spiderwebs are a great holiday motif and are simple to create using straight and curved lines. Orange and black contrast well, but you can also try using different color combinations on each nail for a festive look.

MATERIALS

• Polish palette
• Striping brush

POLISH COLORS

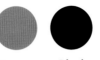

Orange   Black

1

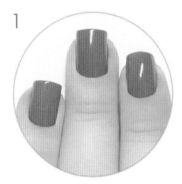

Polish your nails orange.

2

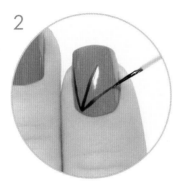

Use your striping brush and black polish or acrylic paint to create three lines at the base of your nail, extending out from the corner.

3

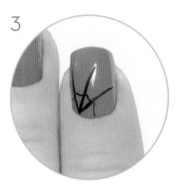

Using your striping brush and black polish or paint, create a small U-shape between each of the lines you made in step 2.

4

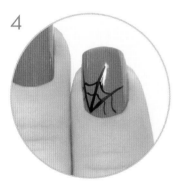

Repeat step 3, moving closer to the ends of the lines. Your U-shapes will be larger than in step 3.

5

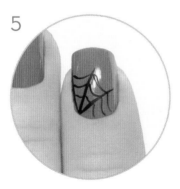

Again, repeat the technique, creating a larger U-shape between each line. Repeat as needed until your web is complete.

6

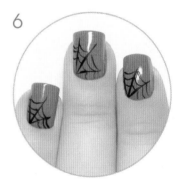

Repeat steps 2 through 5 on all nails, or wear the spiderweb as an accent nail.

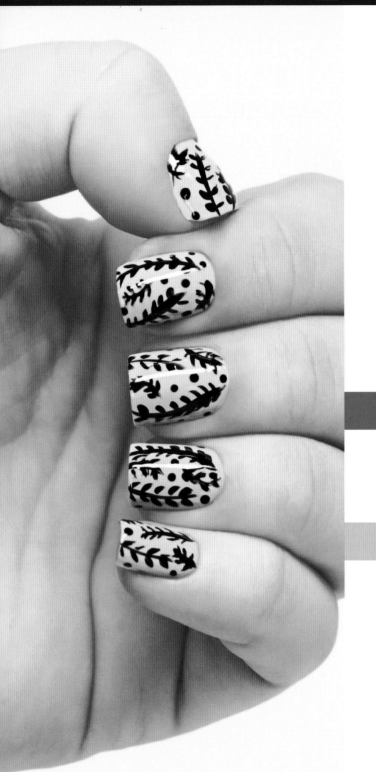

BAROQUE VINES

Abstract vines are a great alternative to floral nails. When done in a navy color scheme, they are reminiscent of fine china. The techniques in this manicure are simple, but you have a lot of creative control in the placement of the vines.

MATERIALS

- Striping brush
- Polish palette
- Dotting tool

POLISH COLORS

Nude   Navy

1

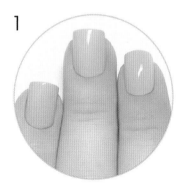

Polish your nails nude.

2

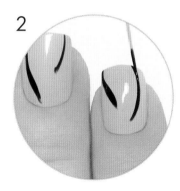

Using your striping brush loaded with navy polish, create one or two long, curved lines on each nail.

3

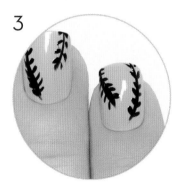

Use short brushstrokes and navy polish to create leaf shapes coming off the lines you created in step 2.

4

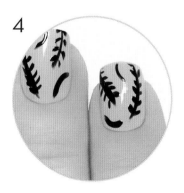

Add some shorter curved lines where there is space on the nail.

5

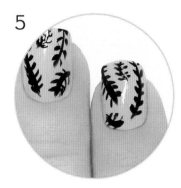

As in step 3, create leaf shapes on the shorter lines.

6

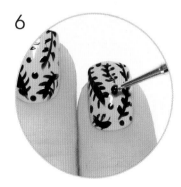

Fill any empty space on the nail with small navy dots.

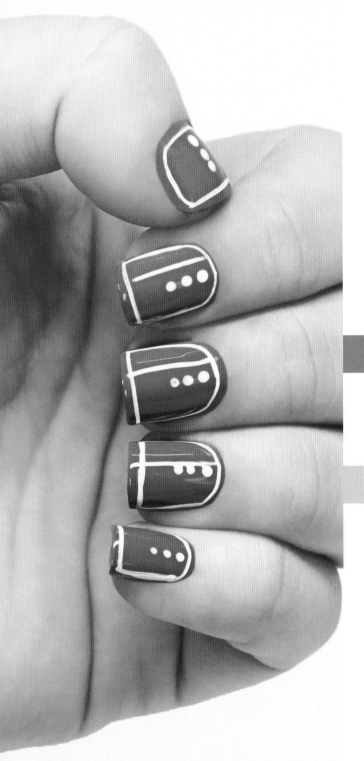

GINGER-BREAD NAILS

This fun holiday manicure turns your nails into an adorable version of the classic Christmas gingerbread cookie. White polish acts as the icing, creating a unique manicure that is sure to get attention.

MATERIALS

• Striping brush
• Polish palette
• Dotting tool

POLISH COLORS

Brown   White

1

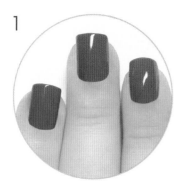

Polish your nails in a brown polish.

2

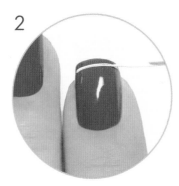

Using your striping brush and white polish or acrylic paint, create a line along the free edge of one nail. Follow the shape of your natural nail.

3

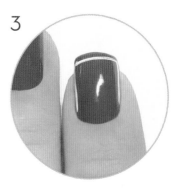

Paint lines near the sidewall on each side of your nail, again following the shape of your nail bed.

4

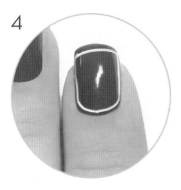

Finish the outline of your nail by following the curve of your cuticle.

5

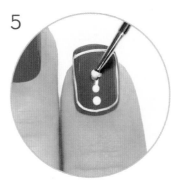

Use the small end of your dotting tool and white polish to create two or three dots from the cuticle, up the center of the nail.

6

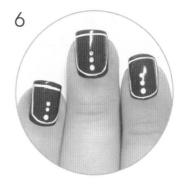

Complete steps 2 through 5 on your other nails.

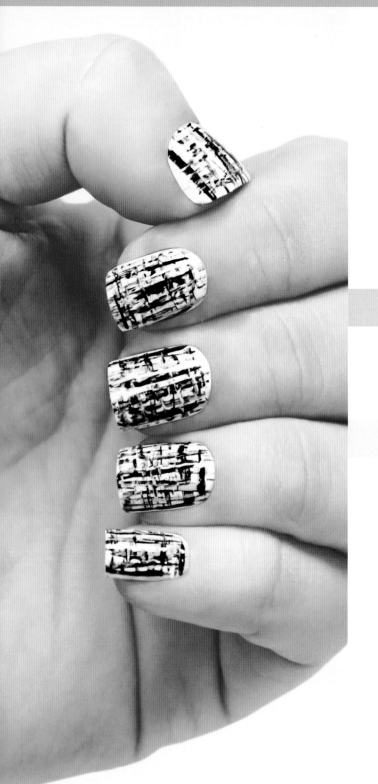

TWEED

Textural manicures are striking and fashion-forward. In this manicure, shades of black and white are layered to create a textile-like finish that goes with anything.

MATERIALS

- Striping brush
- Polish palette
- Paper towel

POLISH COLORS

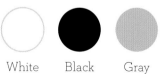

White   Black   Gray

1

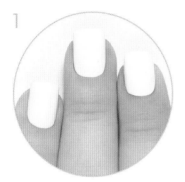

Polish your nails white.
Let dry.

2

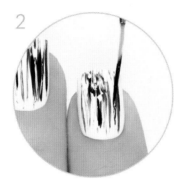

Load your striping brush with
black polish and wipe it off
on a paper towel, leaving a
small amount of polish on
the bristles. Create several
vertical brushstrokes on the
nail.

3

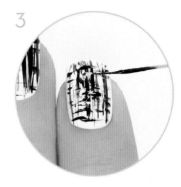

Using the same technique,
create horizontal strokes
across the nail in black.

4

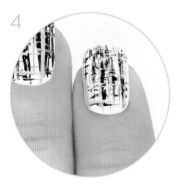

Layer a series of vertical and
horizontal gray brushstrokes
over the black ones.

5

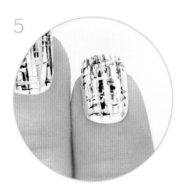

Layer white vertical and
horizontal brushstrokes over
the entire nail.

6

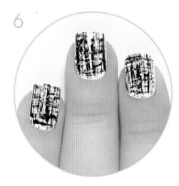

If needed, go back in
with several more black
brushstrokes to create more
depth on the nail.

TAPE TREE

Using stationery tape and striping tape, you can create a crisp Christmas tree manicure without any freehand art. Pair it with polka dots and festive colors for a great holiday look.

MATERIALS

- Stationery tape
- Striping tape
- Dotting tool
- Polish palette

POLISH COLORS

Red   Green   Gold

TAPE

1
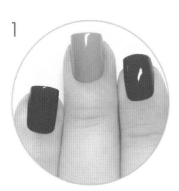

Paint your nails red with a green accent nail on your middle finger. Let dry completely.

2
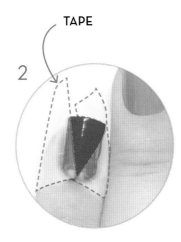

On the ring nail, apply two pieces of tape that come to a point near the base of the nail, leaving a triangle shape exposed.

3
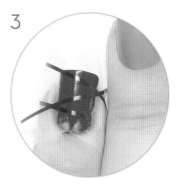

Add three or four pieces of striping tape in a zigzag pattern over the exposed nail.

4
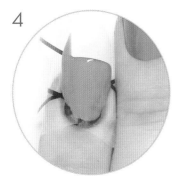

Paint green polish over the exposed part of the nail.

5
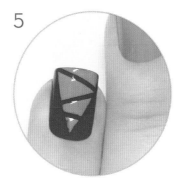

Immediately after applying polish, carefully remove both types of tape.

6
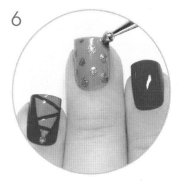

If desired, add a gold dot at the tip of the tree you just created and more gold dots on the green accent nail.

ART DECO TIPS

Artistic black-and-white nails are a classic any time of year. If you are very patient, you could use striping tape to create this design, but this tutorial shows how to create a clean yet organic look using your striping brush.

MATERIALS

• Striping brush
• Polish palette

POLISH COLORS

Black   White

1

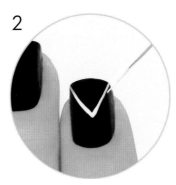

Polish your nails black.

2

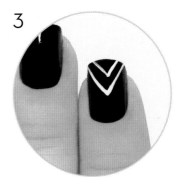

Using your striping brush and white polish or acrylic paint, paint a V-shape on one nail, starting at the free edge and coming to a point in the center of the nail.

3

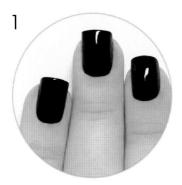

Using the same technique, paint a smaller V-shape within the first one.

4

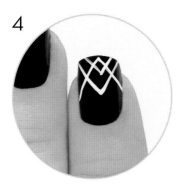

Create a V-shape oriented in the opposite direction, coming to a point within the V from step 3.

5

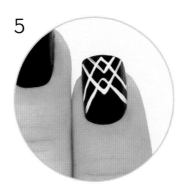

Repeat step 4, starting farther down the nail.

6

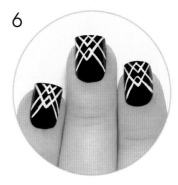

Repeat steps 2 through 5 on the rest of your nails.

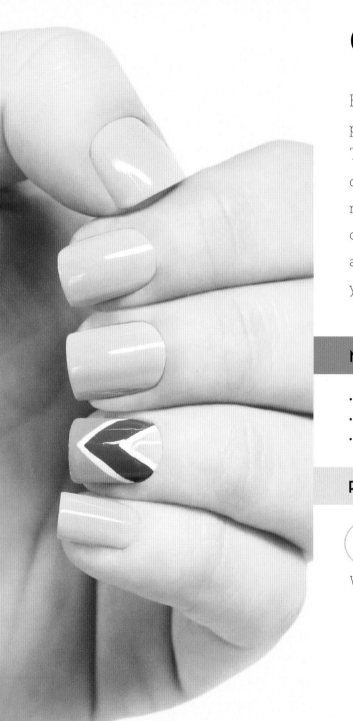

CHEVRONS

Brightly colored chevrons are perfect for a summertime manicure. This design uses striping tape to create crisp white lines that contrast nicely against the bright colors. You can also use the chevron design as an accent nail to add interest to your manicure.

MATERIALS

• Striping tape
• Striping brush
• Polish palette

POLISH COLORS

White Lavender Blue Pink

1

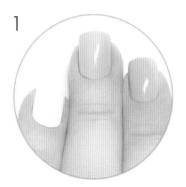

Polish your nails lavender with a white accent nail on your ring finger. Let dry completely.

2

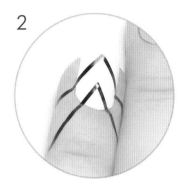

Apply striping tape to the white nail in upward V-shapes, as shown.

3

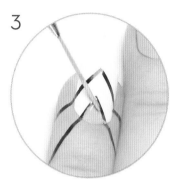

Paint the triangle near the cuticle with lavender polish using your striping brush.

4

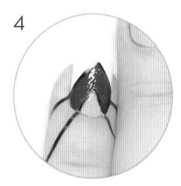

Paint the V-shape in the middle of the nail with blue polish using your striping brush.

5

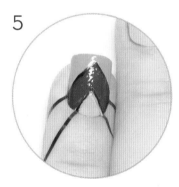

Paint the remaining space near the free edge with pink polish using your striping brush.

6

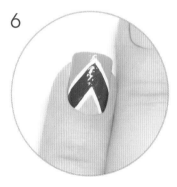

Immediately after polishing, carefully remove the striping tape.

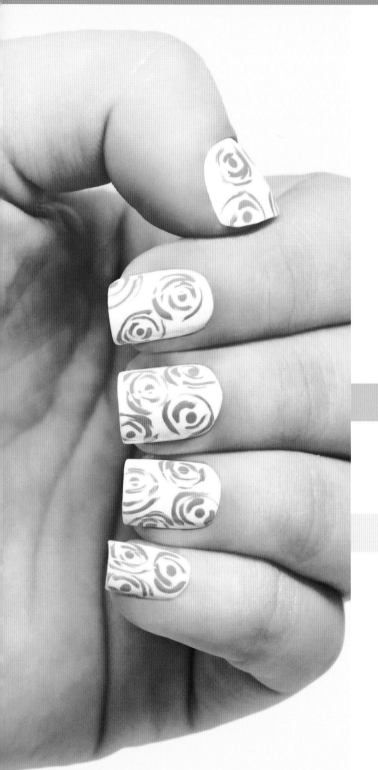

ABSTRACT ROSES

Simple brush strokes and dots come together to create graphic, abstract rose motifs in this manicure. Create several roses in different colors on each nail as shown here, or create one large rose radiating across the entire nail.

MATERIALS

• Dotting tool
• Polish palette
• Striping brush

POLISH COLORS

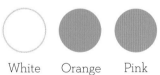

White   Orange   Pink

1

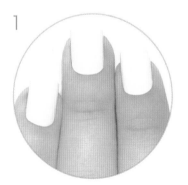

Polish your nails white.

2

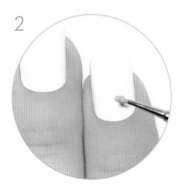

Make a small orange dot on one nail.

3

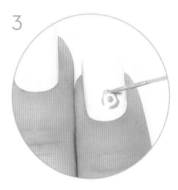

Using your striping brush, create two round shapes around the dot in orange polish.

4

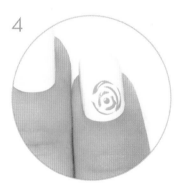

Make several more circular shapes to create a rose.

5

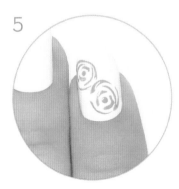

Repeat steps 2 through 4 on the same nail using pink polish.

6

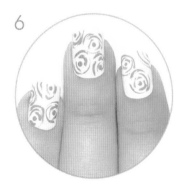

Fill all of your nails with orange and pink roses.

WHIMSICAL FLORAL

This whimsical floral design is great for those who aren't yet confident with detailed free-hand work. Use bright, contrasting shades on a neutral background for an exciting look that is perfect for spring or summer.

MATERIALS

• Dotting tool
• Polish palette
• Striping brush

POLISH COLORS

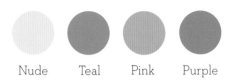

Nude   Teal   Pink   Purple

1

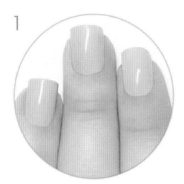

Polish your nails nude.

2

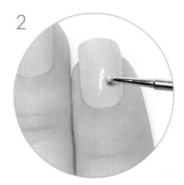

Use your dotting tool to create a small teal dot on one nail.

3

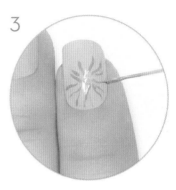

Using your striping brush and pink polish, paint several squiggly lines radiating from the teal dot to create a flower.

4

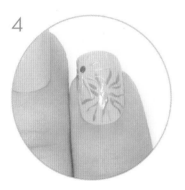

Repeat steps 2 and 3, this time with a purple center and teal squiggles. The squiggles can overlap.

5

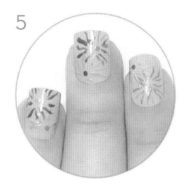

Fill all of your nails with flowers, changing the color combinations as you go.

6

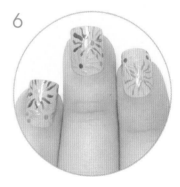

Fill any empty space on the nails with purple, teal, and pink dots.

SIDEWALL MOONS

This monochromatic take on a classic moon manicure features several shades and finishes of pink. For an edgier look, try this manicure in contrasting bold shades.

MATERIALS

- Striping brush
- Polish palette
- Top coat (not quick-dry)
- Dotting tool
- Pink hexangonal glitter

POLISH COLORS

Pink   Metallic pink

1

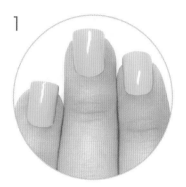

Polish your nails in a pink polish.

2

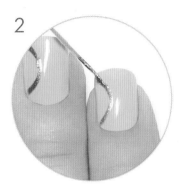

Using your striping brush, create a curved line near the sidewall of each nail in metallic pink polish.

3

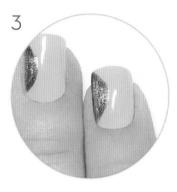

Fill in the half-moon shape using your striping brush and metallic pink polish.

4

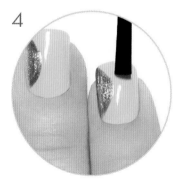

Apply a top coat to one nail.

5

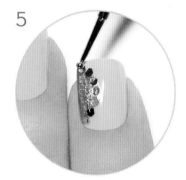

Using a dotting tool dipped in top coat, place pink hexagonal glitter pieces along the border of the half-moon-shape.

6

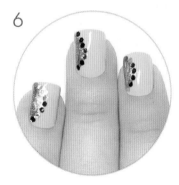

Repeat steps 4 and 5 on all nails. Seal the glitter in with two coats of top coat.

DOT GRADIENT

The Dot Gradient manicure combines a simple dotting technique with countless color combination possibilities. Adapt this manicure for different holidays or seasons by choosing different colors for your dots. Bold purple and blue dots are great for any time of year.

MATERIALS

• Dotting tool
• Polish palette

POLISH COLORS

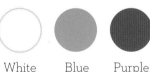

White   Blue   Purple

1

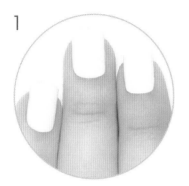

Polish your nails white.

2

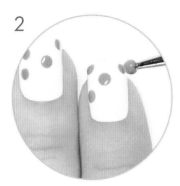

Using a dotting tool and blue polish, create several large dots on the half of the nail closest to the free edge.

3

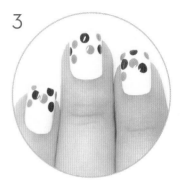

Add several purple dots to the same area. They can overlap the blue dots.

4

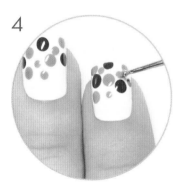

Using the small end of your dotting tool, add small blue dots that overlap the other dots.

5

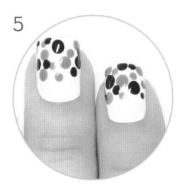

Repeat step 4 with small purple dots.

6

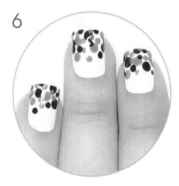

Create more dots to fill in the nail closest to the free edge, creating a gradient effect.

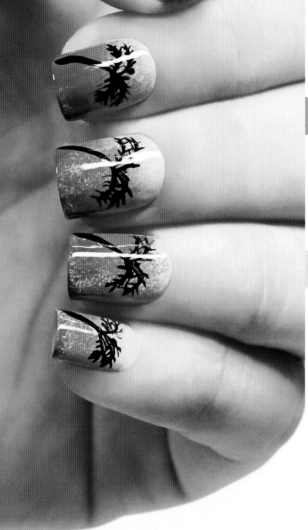

PALM TREES

Jetting off on a tropical vacation? This manicure is perfect for that, or for any time you need to achieve a beach bum state of mind. The gradient and palm tree silhouettes evoke images of sunsets over the warm ocean.

MATERIALS

- Cosmetic sponge
- Acetone
- Clean-up brush
- Striping brush
- Polish palette
- Top coat

POLISH COLORS

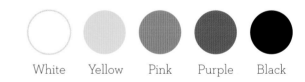

White   Yellow   Pink   Purple   Black

1

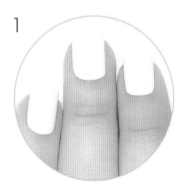

Polish your nails white. Let dry completely.

2

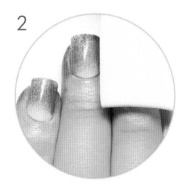

Paint stripes of yellow, pink, and purple polish on a cosmetic sponge and stamp it onto each nail.

3

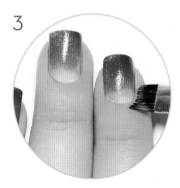

Repeat step 2 until the gradient is vibrant. Clean up with acetone and angled eyeliner brush.

4

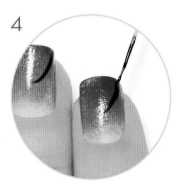

Using your black striping brush and black polish or acrylic paint, paint a curved line from the center of your nail to one corner of the free edge.

5

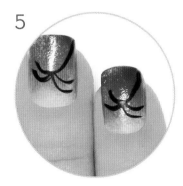

Use your striping brush to create the branches of the palm tree.

6

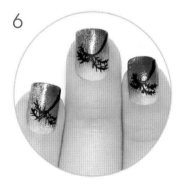

Add short thin lines off of each branch until the palm tree is complete. Seal the design with top coat.

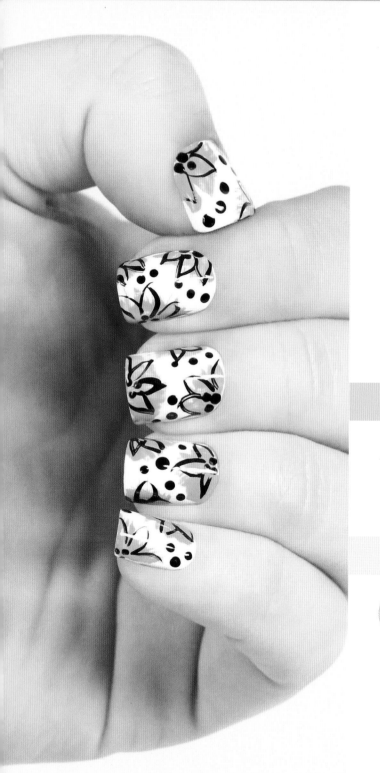

SPRING FLOWERS

These bright spring flowers play up the contrast between black and white with splashes of color. Use flowing strokes of your striping brush to create artistic flowers all over your nails. For a bolder look, use multiple colors to make the splashes.

MATERIALS

• Striping brush
• Polish palette
• Dotting tool

POLISH COLORS

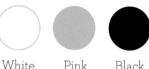

White   Pink   Black

1

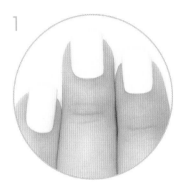

Polish your nails with a white polish.

2

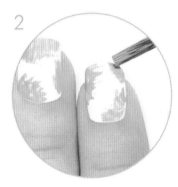

Use your polish brush to paint messy pink "splashes" of color all over your nails. For a complete look, create some partial splashes at the edges of your nails.

3

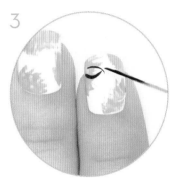

Using your striping brush and black polish or acrylic paint, create a petal shape on top of one of the pink splashes.

4

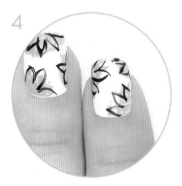

Use a similar technique to create four- or five-petal flowers on top of each splash.

5

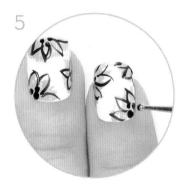

Use your dotting tool and black polish to add two or three dots to the center of each flower.

6

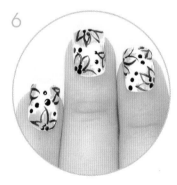

Fill any empty space on your nail with black dots.

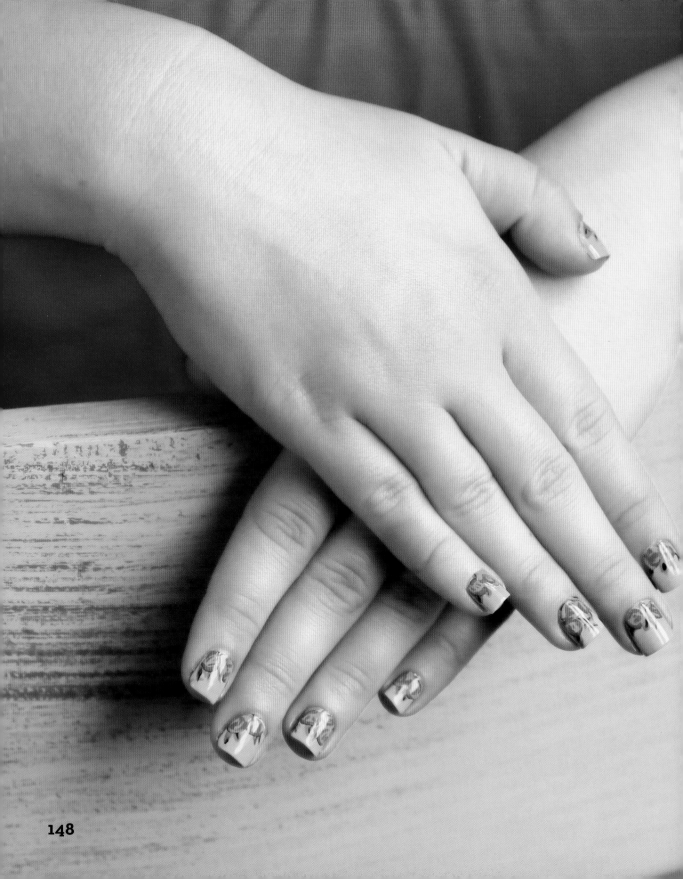

ADVANCED DESIGNS

The advanced manicures in this section feature beautiful freehand designs, as well as more complex applications of the basic techniques you have learned so far. Many of these tutorials require some artistic interpretation, so have fun and express yourself with confidence. As with the previous tutorials in this book, these manicures can be adapted for any occasion with different polish shades and finishes.

ZIGZAGS

Zigzag manicures can be extremely bold with contrasting shades, or chic with soft, feminine polishes. When you start with a well-spaced grid, your zigzags will spread evenly across your nails.

MATERIALS

• Striping brush
• Polish palette

POLISH COLORS

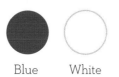

Blue   White

1

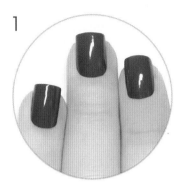

Polish your nails blue.

2

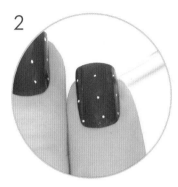

Use the tip of your striping brush and white polish to make a grid of tiny dots across your nails.

3

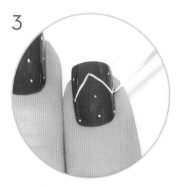

Using your striping brush and white polish or acrylic paint, connect the dots in a zigzag pattern.

4

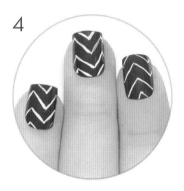

Continue to paint zigzags on your nails until all of the dots of the grids are connected.

5

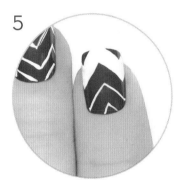

Use your striping brush and white polish to fill in the space between two of the zigzag lines.

6

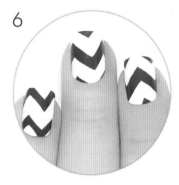

Continue to fill in zigzags, alternating white and blue.

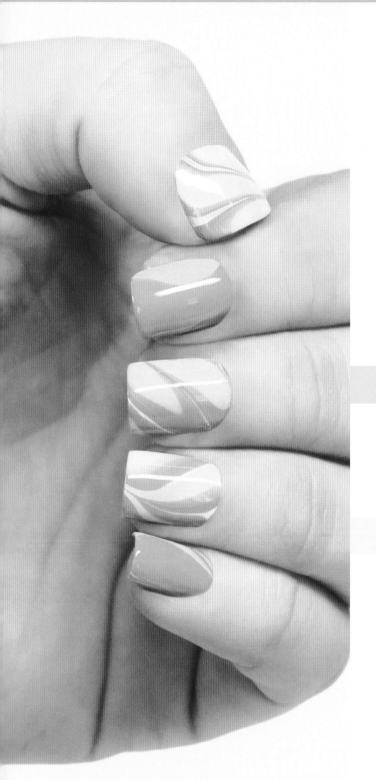

WATER MARBLE

The water marble technique may be daunting, but the finished look is well worth the time and patience it takes. Endless color combinations and designs can be created, and like most things, practice makes perfect.

MATERIALS

- Paper towels
- Small cup
- Water
- Tape
- Toothpicks
- Acetone
- Clean-up brush

POLISH COLORS

White   Pink   Gray   Blue

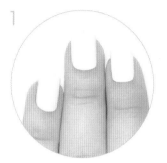

1

Prepare your work area by laying down paper towels if needed. Paint your nails white. Let dry completely.

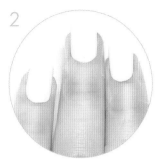

2

Fill a small cup with room-temperature filtered or bottled water. Apply tape around your nails to ease clean up.

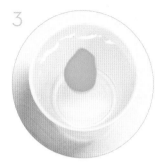

3

Holding the polish brush over the cup, place a drop of pink polish onto the surface of the water, allowing it to spread out.

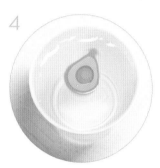

4

Carefully place three to four more drops of polish on top of the first drop. Allow each color to spread out before adding the next drop.

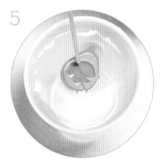

5

Drag the tip of a toothpick through the polish on the surface of the water, creating the desired design or swirls.

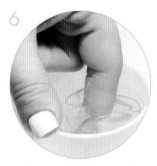

6

Angle your finger so that the nail is parallel to the surface of the water and carefully dip one nail through the polish. Hold it under water until the polish dries.

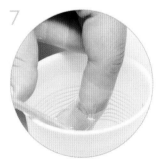

7

Use a toothpick to remove the excess dried polish on the surface of the water.

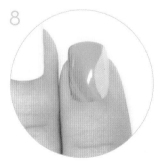

8

Carefully remove your finger from the water. Remove the tape and use acetone and an angled eyeliner brush to clean up.

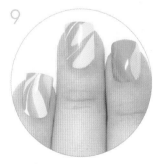

9

Repeat steps 3 through 8 on the rest of your nails, or wear a water marble as an accent nail.

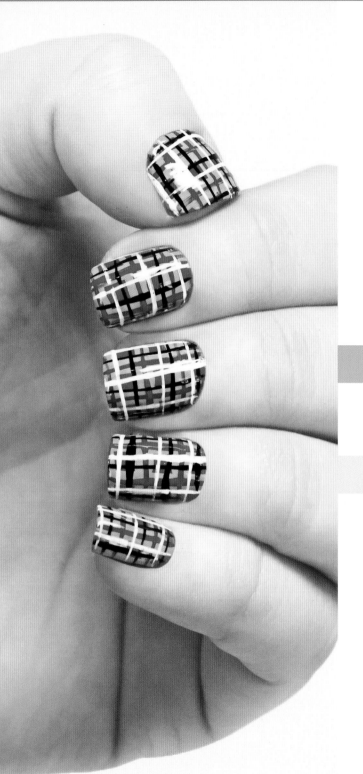

PLAID

While the plaid manicure appears to be complex, it is actually just a layering of simple straight lines. Take it one step at a time. Try this festive red and green color scheme, or use one of your favorite color combinations.

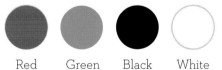

1

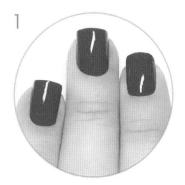

Polish your nails red.

2

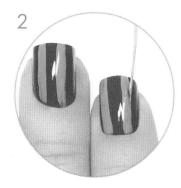

Using your striping brush and green polish, paint several thick vertical lines on your nails.

3

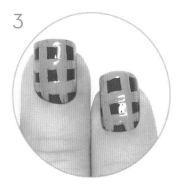

Paint several thick horizontal green stripes, creating a series of red squares across your nails.

4

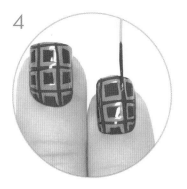

Use your striping brush and red polish to paint thin lines on top of the thick green ones.

5

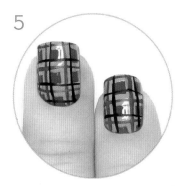

Paint a grid of thin black lines, slightly to the right and above the red lines.

6

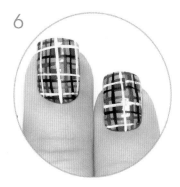

Paint a grid of thin white lines, slightly to the right and above the black ones. Finish the look with a top coat.

GALAXY

The Galaxy manicure is a classic technique that puts the cosmos at your fingertips. By layering colors with a sponge and adding lots of sparkle, you can create impressively complex galaxy designs.

MATERIALS

- Shimmer top coat
- Cosmetic sponge
- Dotting tool
- Polish palette
- Glitter polish

POLISH COLORS

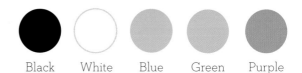

Black   White   Blue   Green   Purple

1

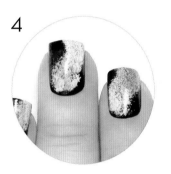

Polish your nails black.

2

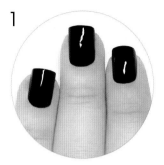

Apply a shimmer top coat over the black polish and let dry completely.

3

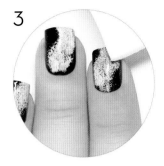

Use a cosmetic sponge to apply a textured band of white polish across each nail. Do not cover the whole nail.

4

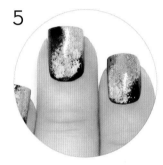

Use a cosmetic sponge to apply some blue polish over the white areas.

5

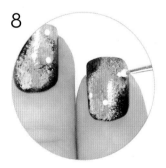

Repeat step 4 with green polish, filling in more of the white space.

6

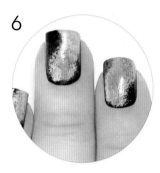

Fill in the remainder of the white space by sponging purple polish onto the nails.

7

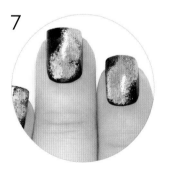

If needed, sponge some black polish around the colors you just added to define the shape of your galaxies.

8

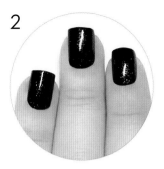

Using a small dotting tool and white polish, apply a few "stars" to your nails. Allow to dry.

9

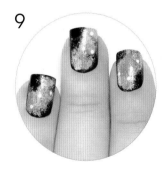

Finish with a sponging of a fine glitter polish to add the perfect amount of sparkle.

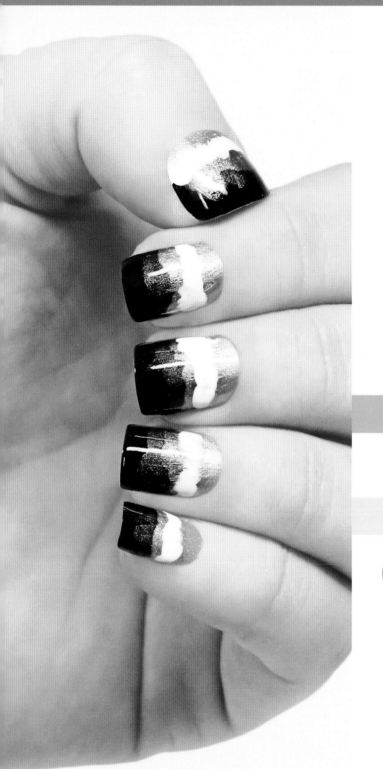

BEACH WAVES

This abstract nature-inspired manicure is reminiscent of the view of the ocean from above. Be creative when you apply the strokes of polish to create a flowing gradient of blues and teals, complete with breaking waves at the coastline.

MATERIALS

• Top coat

POLISH COLORS

| Gold | Navy blue | Blue metallic | Teal | White |

1

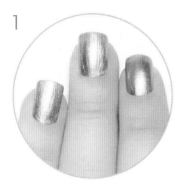

Paint your nails gold and let dry.

2

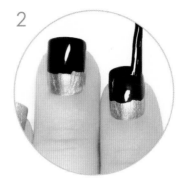

Using the brush from the bottle, apply a thin coat of navy polish from halfway down the nail to the free edge.

3

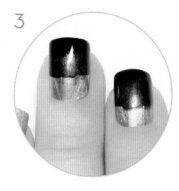

Paint over the lower half of the navy section in blue metallic polish. Use irregular strokes to create the look of shallower water close to the gold "sand."

4

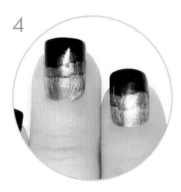

Using the same technique, apply a layer of teal polish overlapping the blue and covering some of the gold.

5

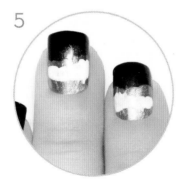

Add a few short brush strokes of white polish where the blue and gold colors meet to represent the breaking waves.

6

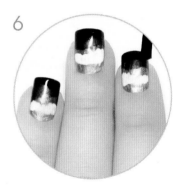

Apply a top coat to blend the colors together slightly and complete the look.

ANGULAR MOONS

This manicure requires an extremely steady hand, but the finished product is worth the time and focus. For detailed work like this, acrylic paint works best since it dries quickly and stays exactly where you apply it.

MATERIALS

• Striping brush
• Polish palette

POLISH COLORS

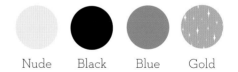

Nude   Black   Blue   Gold

1

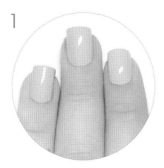

Paint your nails nude and
let dry.

2

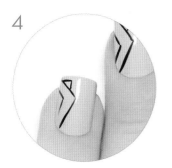

Using a striping brush and
black polish or acrylic paint,
make a V-shape coming from
the sidewall of each nail.

3

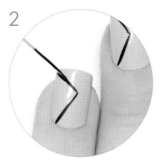

Paint a second V-shape within
the first one, closer to the
sidewall.

4

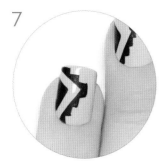

Carefully paint a small right
angle coming off the V-shape
you made in step 2.

5

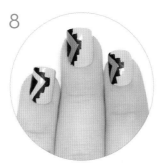

Repeat step 4, adding right
angles around the entire
V-shape on all of your nails.

6

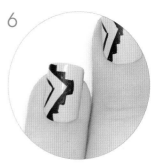

Carefully use your striping
brush to fill in the angles with
black polish or acrylic paint.

7

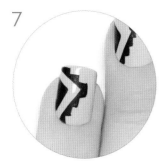

Fill in the space between the
sidewall and smallest V-shape
with black polish or acrylic
paint.

8

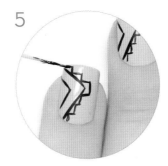

On all of your nails except
your ring finger, fill in the final
V-shape with blue polish.

9

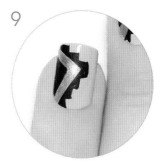

Create an accent nail by
filling in the final V-shape
on your ring finger with gold
polish.

SUGAR SKULLS

This manicure uses several techniques to create a fun sugar skull design. Whether you wear this as an accent nail or sport ten little skulls, it's sure to be noticed.

MATERIALS

- Striping brush
- Polish palette
- Dotting tool

POLISH COLORS

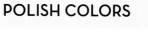

Pink   White   Black   Yellow

Orange   Blue

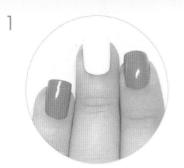

1

Paint your nails pink with a white accent nail.

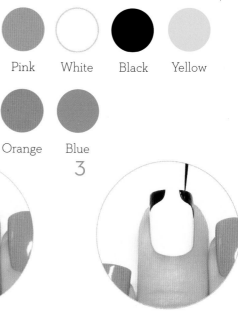

2

Use a striping brush and black polish to create two curved lines on accent nail, from the sidewall to the free edge, creating a jawline.

3

Fill in the space you created in step 2 with black polish.

4

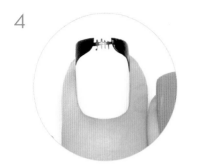

Use your striping brush and black polish to paint a line with hash marks along it, creating a mouth.

5

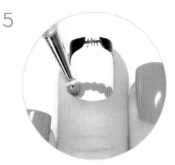

Use a dotting tool and pink polish to create a semicircle of overlapping dots near the base of the nail.

6

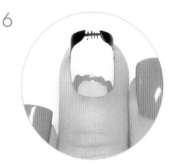

Use your dotting tool to fill in the space between the pink dots and the base of the nail with yellow polish.

7

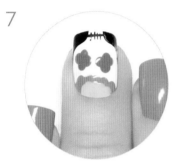

Use your dotting tool and orange polish to create two sets of four overlapping dots in a cross shape.

8

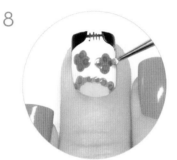

Using a small dotting tool and blue polish, add small accent dots to the pink and orange dots.

9

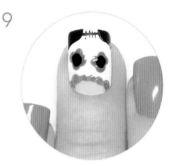

Add the eye sockets to the skulls with black polish and a dotting tool.

10

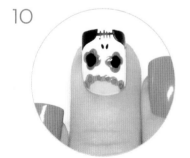

Use a striping brush and black polish to paint two angled lines, creating a nose.

11

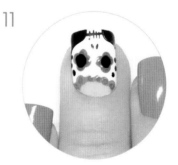

Using a small dotting tool and black polish, add a few accent dots on the outside of the eyes.

12

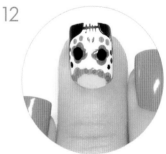
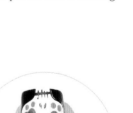

Add a few pink accent dots where the cheekbones would be.

JACK-O-LANTERN

You can't go wrong with jack-o-lantern nails for Halloween. This tutorial shows you how to create a traditional jack-o-lantern accent nail, but you can be creative with the shape of the eyes and mouth to create a unique face.

MATERIALS

- Striping brush
- Polish palette

POLISH COLORS

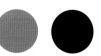

Orange   Black

1

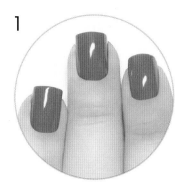

Polish your nails orange.

2

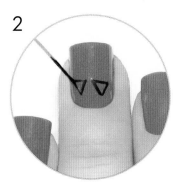

Use your striping brush and black polish or acrylic paint to create two small triangles. These are the jack-o-lantern's eyes.

3

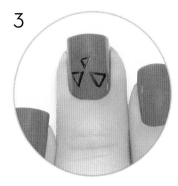

Paint a third, smaller triangle centered on the nail. This is the jack-o-lantern's nose.

4

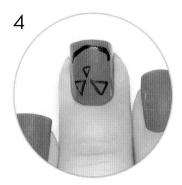

Create the beginning of the mouth by painting a curved line near your free edge.

5

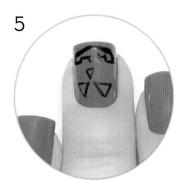

Finish the mouth with a notched line across the top.

6

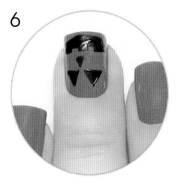

Fill in the shapes you created in the previous steps with black polish or acrylic paint.

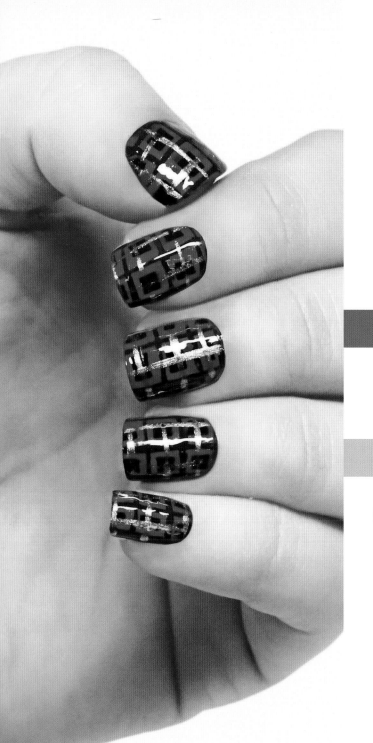

TARTAN

This variation on a plaid manicure is perfectly sophisticated and great for the holidays! Once you have mastered basic stripes, this manicure will be well within your skill set.

MATERIALS

- Striping brush
- Polish palette

POLISH COLORS

| Navy | Red | Red metallic | Dark green | Gold |

1

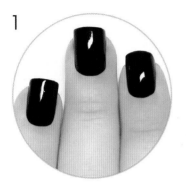

Polish your nails navy blue.

2

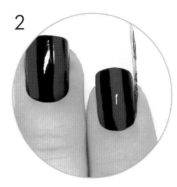

Using a striping brush, paint thick vertical stripes in a red polish. Evenly space them across your nail.

3

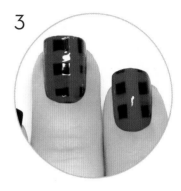

Using the same method, create thick red horizontal stripes that overlap the vertical ones.

4

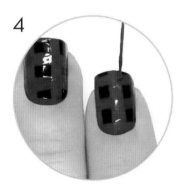

Where the red stripes overlap, paint metallic red squares with your striping brush to add shimmer to the design.

5

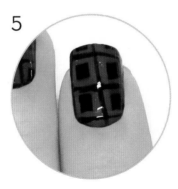

Again using a striping brush, paint thin dark green stripes centered over the thick red stripes.

6

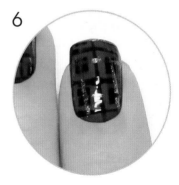

Paint thin gold stripes centered over the space between the red stripes.

SAFARI NAILS

This manicure combines three phenomenal nail art techniques: sponging, leopard, and zebra. They come together to create a playfully wild design. This tutorial features bright shades, but you could use earth tones for a more natural look.

MATERIALS

• Cosmetic sponge
• Striping brush
• Polish palette
• Dotting tool

POLISH COLORS

Yellow   Pink   Black

1

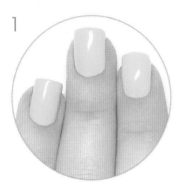

Polish your nails in yellow polish. Let dry.

2

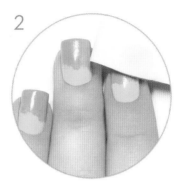

Use a cosmetic sponge to add some pink polish to the tips of your nails. This does not need to be perfect.

3

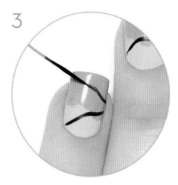

Using your striping brush and black polish or acrylic paint, make two squiggly lines coming to a point near the sidewall.

4

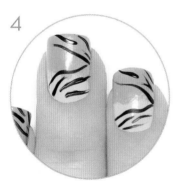

Create several more zebra stripes, filling in the spaces near the free edge and the base of the nail.

5

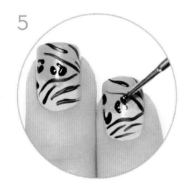

Use your dotting tool and black polish to create small leopard spots in the remaining space. C-shapes work well.

6

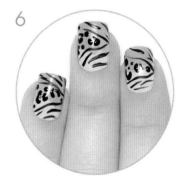

Fill in the empty space left on your nails with small black dots.

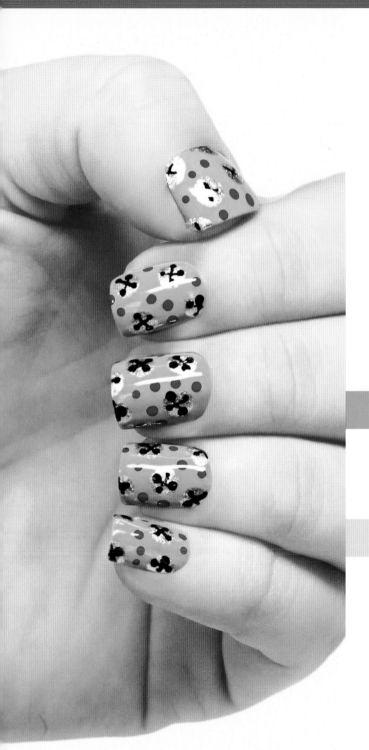

JINGLE BELLS

This holiday manicure is perfectly festive. The contrast of metallic and crème polishes and the detail of the bells make for an interesting design that can be used on all ten nails or as an accent nail.

MATERIALS

- Dotting tool
- Polish palette
- Striping brush

POLISH COLORS

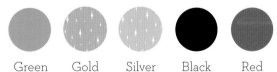

Green   Gold   Silver   Black   Red

1

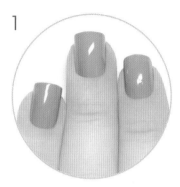

Polish your nails green.

2

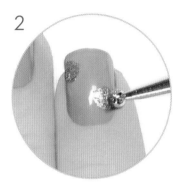

Use your dotting tool and gold polish to make several large dots, spread across your nails.

3

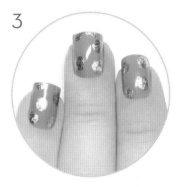

Use the same technique to create several large silver dots.

4

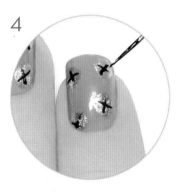

Use your striping brush and black polish or acrylic paint to make a small "+" shape on each circle.

5

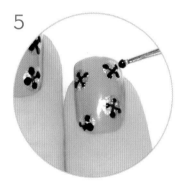

Use the small end of your dotting tool and black polish to add tiny dots to the ends of each "+" sign.

6

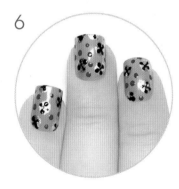

Fill in the remaining space on each nail with red dots.

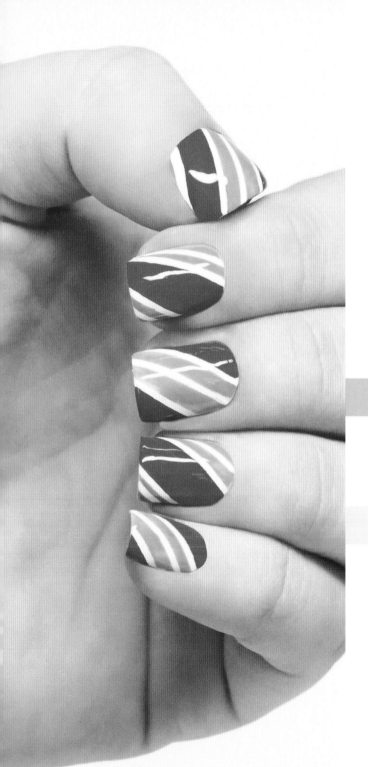

CANDY CANES

Striping tape and holiday polish colors come together in this Christmas manicure. You could use your striping brush to paint these stripes, but the tape creates crisp lines in red and green to emulate a tasty holiday treat.

MATERIALS

- Striping tape
- Striping brush
- Polish palette

POLISH COLORS

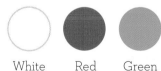

White   Red   Green

1

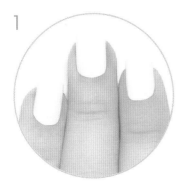

Paint your nails white. Let dry completely.

2

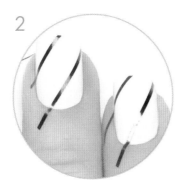

Apply striping tape to your nails on a diagonal, spread widely across the nail plate.

3

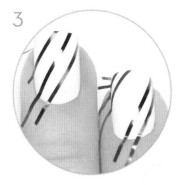

Add another piece of striping tape between the pieces you placed in step 2. Do this between every other piece.

4

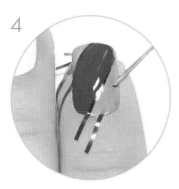

On one nail, paint red polish over the widely spaced tape and green over the sections with two pieces of tape.

5

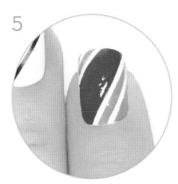

Immediately after polishing, carefully remove the tape.

6

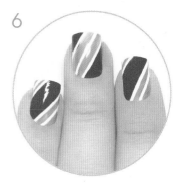

Complete steps 4 and 5 on the rest of your nails, one nail at a time.

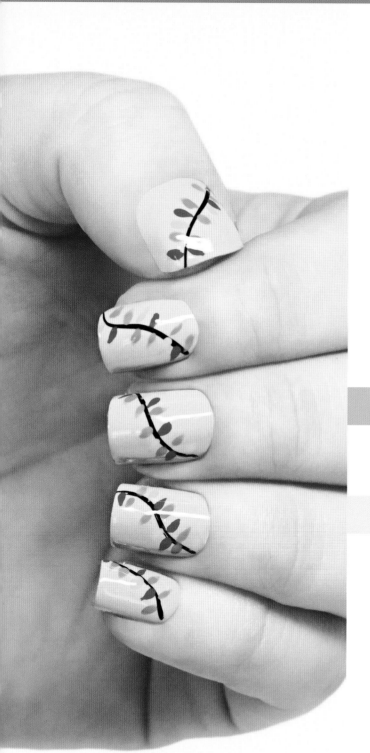

HOLIDAY LIGHTS

This colorful holiday manicure uses strokes of your striping brush to create a string of lights across your nails. Use this design on its own or as one element in a Christmas manicure with the other holiday designs from this book.

MATERIALS

• Striping brush
• Polish palette

POLISH COLORS

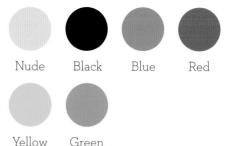

Nude   Black   Blue   Red

Yellow   Green

1

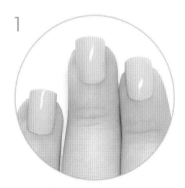

Paint your nails nude.

2

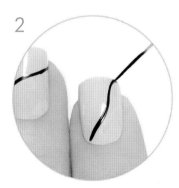

Use your striping brush and black polish or acrylic paint to create a curved line across each nail.

3

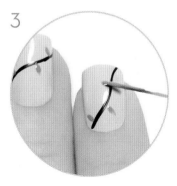

Use you striping brush to add small light bulb shapes along the black line in blue polish.

4

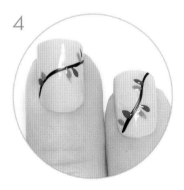

Using a similar technique, add red light bulbs.

5

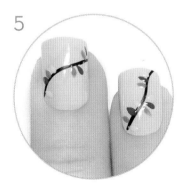

Add more bulbs, this time in yellow polish.

6

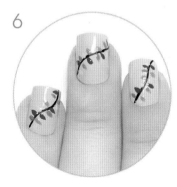

Complete the string of lights with green bulbs, and fill in any remaining space with colors of your choice.

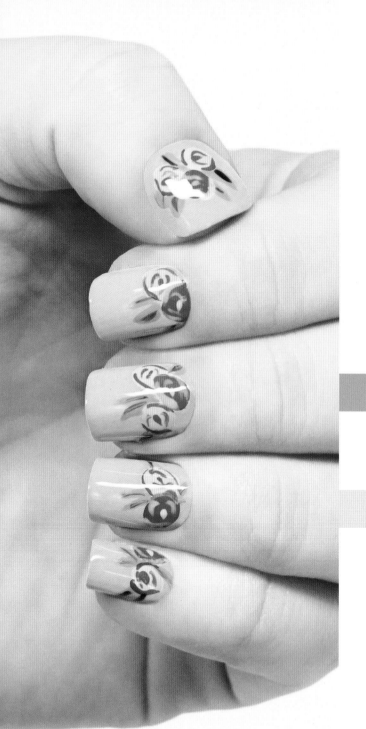

DETAILED ROSES

There are few nail art designs more feminine than flowers. Soft details along with multiple shades of pink and green bring roses to life on your nails. The bold teal base color pops against the pinks of the flowers.

MATERIALS

• Striping brush
• Polish palette

POLISH COLORS

| Teal | Light pink | Dark pink | Light green | Dark green |

1

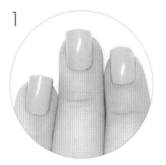

Polish your nails teal.

2

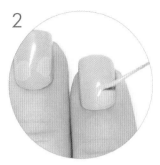

Use your striping brush to paint one or two circular shapes in light pink polish near the base of each nail.

3

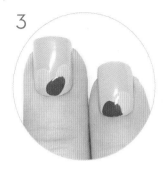

Add a dark pink circular shape to each nail, creating clusters of roses.

4

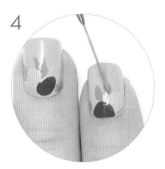

Use your striping brush and light green polish to paint several triangular leaves on each cluster of roses.

5

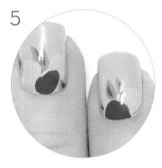

Use your striping brush and dark green polish to add a short detail line down the center of each leaf.

6

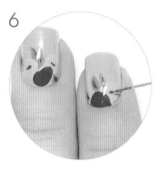

Use your striping brush and dark pink polish to add a small dot mark at the center of each light pink rose.

7

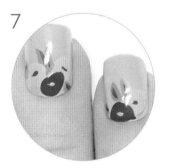

Repeat step 6, this time placing light pink dot marks in each dark pink rose.

8

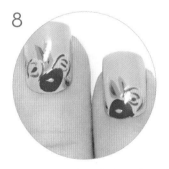

Use dark pink polish and your striping brush to add subtle detail to the light pink roses. Round shapes work well.

9

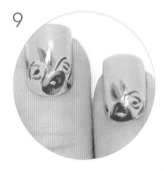

Repeat step 8, using light pink polish to add detail to the dark pink roses.

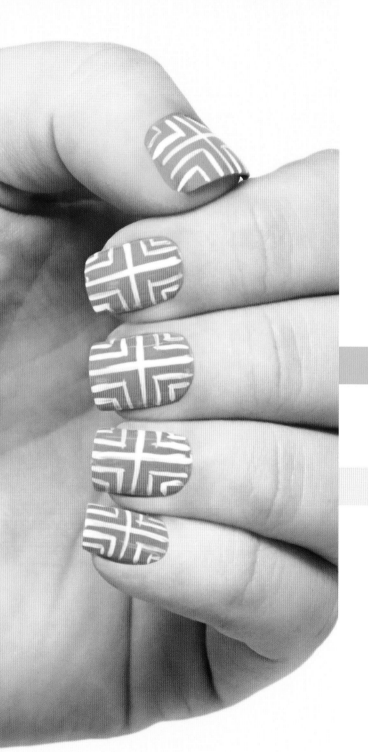

CRISSCROSS

This graphic manicure brings together short line segments to create an eye-catching design. The neon pink polish used here is perfect for summertime, but you could change up the color scheme of this design to fit any season or holiday.

MATERIALS

• Striping brush
• Polish palette

POLISH COLORS

Neon pink

White

1

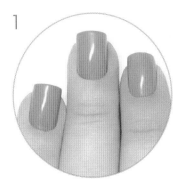

Paint your nails neon pink. Let dry.

2

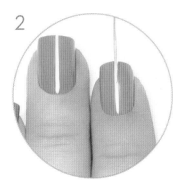

Use your striping brush and white polish or acrylic paint to make a vertical line down the center of each nail.

3

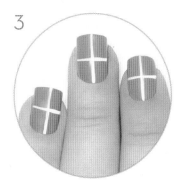

Paint a white horizontal line on each nail, creating a cross shape.

4

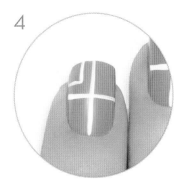

In one of the quadrants created by the cross, paint two small line segments, following the shape of the original lines.

5

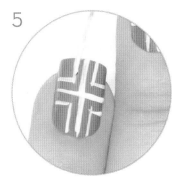

Continue to fill in quadrants of the manicure with line segments using white polish or acrylic paint.

6

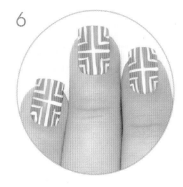

If the size of your nails permits, add another set of lines to each nail.

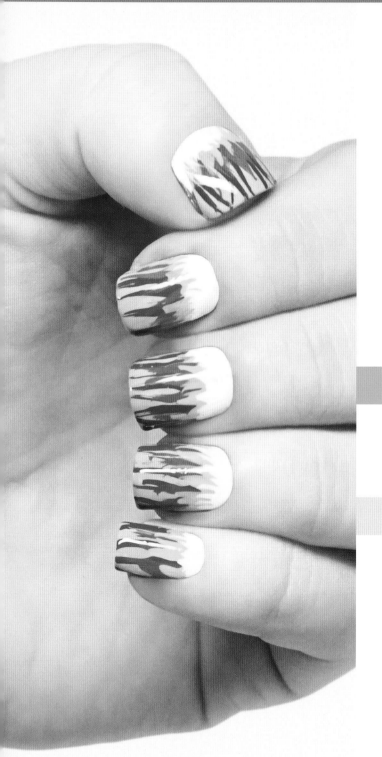

FIRE MANICURE

Flames on your nails make for a feisty and fun manicure. This tutorial outlines a fiery red flame, but you could also do this in a cool color scheme to create a unique gradient look.

MATERIALS

• Striping brush
• Polish palette
• Top coat

POLISH COLORS

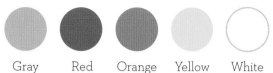

Gray   Red   Orange   Yellow   White

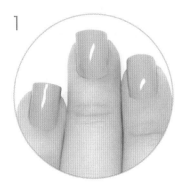

1

Paint your nails gray.

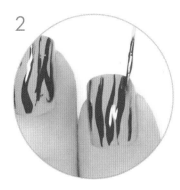

2

Use your striping brush and red polish to create a series of brushstrokes across most of the nail.

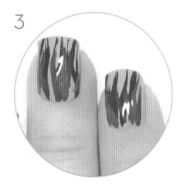

3

Use your striping brush and orange polish to add orange brushstrokes, leaving some red exposed near the free edge.

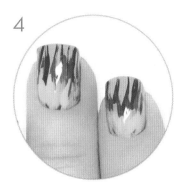

4

Using a similar technique, apply some yellow brush-strokes to your nail, closer to the base.

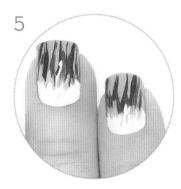

5

Finish the "fire" gradient with some short white brushstrokes at the very base of your nail.

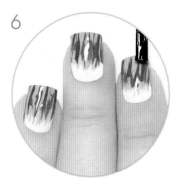

6

Apply a top coat to smooth the colors of the fire gradient.

UNION JACK

Flags can make for great nail art inspiration, as they are colorful and graphic. The Union Jack makes a great nail art design with its angles and contrasting colors. Wear this design as an accent nail with a classy red manicure.

MATERIALS

• Striping brush
• Polish palette

POLISH COLORS

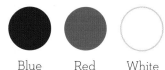

Blue   Red   White

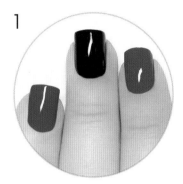

1

Polish your nails red with a blue accent nail. Let dry.

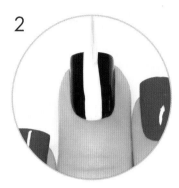

2

Using your striping brush and white polish, paint a thick white line vertically down the center of your accent nail.

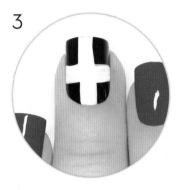

3

Paint a thick white horizontal line across the center of your nail, creating a cross shape.

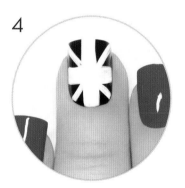

4

Use your striping brush and white polish to paint an X-shape over the cross. These lines should be slightly thinner.

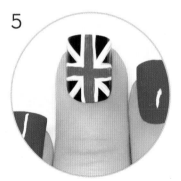

5

Use your striping brush and red polish to paint a red cross layered over the white one. Leave a white border on either side of the lines.

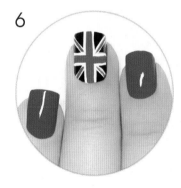

6

Finish with thin red lines layered over the white X-shape. Leave a white border on either side and between the red X-shape and the cross.

BULL'S-EYE DOTS

This manicure is made up of layered dots that create a bull's-eye pattern. Take your time to let the dots dry so the polish does not get too thick. As always, get creative with your color choices; the possibilities are endless.

MATERIALS

• Dotting tool
• Polish palette

POLISH COLORS

White   Blue   Red

1

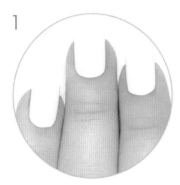

Paint your nails white and let dry.

2

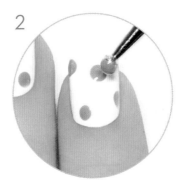

Use your dotting tool to create blue dots, placed randomly across your nails.

3

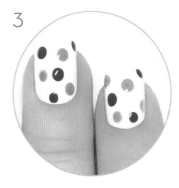

Use your dotting tool and red polish to add some red dots, placed randomly on the nails.

4

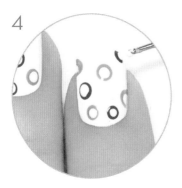

Use the small end of your dotting tool to place white dots in the center of all of the red and blue dots you created.

5

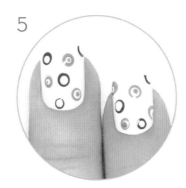

Using the small end of your dotting tool, carefully create tiny blue dots in the center of the blue dots with white centers.

6

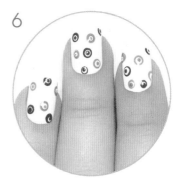

Repeat step 5, this time with red polish on the red dots with white centers.

APPENDIX A:

GLOSSARY

3-FREE Term used to describe a product that does not include formaldehyde, toluene, or dibutyl phthalate.

5-FREE Term used to describe a product that does not include formaldehyde, toluene, dibutyl phthalate, camphor, or formaldehyde resin.

ACCENT NAIL One or two nails polished differently than the other nails in a manicure.

ACETONE Strong solvent used to remove nail polish and soak-off gel manicures.

BASE COAT A clear coat applied to the nail to prevent staining and help with polish adhesion.

BIG 3 A group of potentially harmful chemicals including formaldehyde, toluene, and dibutyl phthalate.

BUFFER A high-grit file used to smooth the nail plate.

CAMPHOR A potentially irritating chemical.

CLEAN-UP BRUSH An angled eyeliner brush used to remove excess polish from the skin.

COSMETIC SPONGE A disposable sponge wedge that can be used to apply polish.

CUTICLE see True Cuticle.

CUTICLE NIPPER A manicure tool used to remove dead tissue from the nail plate.

CUTICLE OIL A mixture of moisturizing oils used on the nail and surrounding skin.

CUTICLE PUSHER A manicure tool used to gently scrape dead cuticle tissue from the nail plate.

CUTICLE REMOVER A cream or gel that contains chemicals that dissolve dead skin from the nail plate.

DEHYDRATOR A product used to dry the nail plate in preparation for a soak-off gel manicure.

DIBUTYL PHTHALATE (DBP) One of the Big 3 chemicals.

DOTTING TOOL Nail art tool with a round end that creates a dot when pressed to the nail.

EPONYCHIUM Living tissue at the base of the nail that creates a seal with the skin.

FILE An abrasive tool used to remove length and shape the free edge of the nail.

FOIL METHOD A method used to remove glitter polish and soak-off gel manicures that involves wrapping the fingertips in foil with a cotton ball soaked in acetone.

FOOT FILE An abrasive tool used to smooth rough, dead skin on the feet.

FORMALDEHYDE One of the Big 3 chemicals.

FORMALDEHYDE RESIN A potentially irritating chemical.

FREE EDGE The part of the nail that grows beyond the fingertip.

HAND CREAM Moisturizing cream or lotion used on the hands and arms.

HYPONYCHIUM Living tissue under the free edge of the nail that creates a seal with the skin.

JOJOBA OIL A natural oil that can penetrate the nail plate.

KERATIN A protein that makes up the hair, skin, and nails.

LANULA The white, moon-shaped part of the nail matrix that is visible under the nail plate.

LATERAL FOLD Living tissue that creates a seal on the sidewall of the nail with the skin.

LED LAMP An electric lamp used to cure soak-off gel manicures.

MANICURE The act of caring for and beautifying the hands and fingernails.

NAIL ADHESIVE Glue used to adhere 3D elements to the nail plate.

NAIL ART TWEEZERS Tweezers with a bent, elongated end used to apply 3D elements to the nail plate.

NAIL CHARM 3D element in any shape that can be applied to the nail plate.

NAIL CLIPPER A manicure tool used to remove length from the free edge of the nail.

NAIL FOIL Metallic foil on a clear backing.

NAIL MATRIX The living portion of the nail where new cells are created.

NAIL PLATE The hard portion of the nail that is polished.

NAIL TREATMENT A clear, brush-on product that contains proteins or chemicals to encourage nail strength and growth.

PEDICURE The art of caring for and beautifying the feet and toenails.

POLISH PALETTE A piece of stiff material such as a paper plate, index card, or foil used to hold puddles of polish for nail art.

SCRUB An abrasive cream or gel that exfoliates the hands or feet.

SHEA BUTTER Natural butter with healing and moisturizing qualities.

SIDEWALL The left and right edges of the nails.

SKITTLE MANICURE A manicure in which each nail is painted with a different color or pattern.

SOAK-OFF GEL A type of nail color that is cured under a UV or LED lamp and requires soaking in acetone for removal.

STATIONERY TAPE Regular invisible tape that can be used in nail art.

STRIPING BRUSH A long, thin paintbrush used for nail art.

STRIPING TAPE Thin tape that is designed specifically for creating crisp lines in nail art.

STUD A small, flat-backed metallic 3D element that can be attached to the nail plate.

TOLUENE One of the Big 3 chemicals.

TOP COAT A clear, brush-on product that helps protect your manicure and add shine.

TRUE CUTICLE The dead, sticky white tissue that forms on your nail plate.

UV LAMP An electric lamp used to cure soak-off gel manicures.

WHITENING SOAK Store-bought or homemade soak used to remove stains from the nail plate.

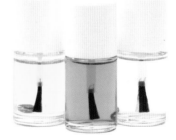

RESOURCES

In this section, you will find resources to help you navigate the world of nail art. There are plenty of websites, blogs, and magazines full of information and inspiration! Also included here is a list of retailers that carry the products used in this book, as well as some of the top brands for nail art and nail care supplies.

WEBSITES Find inspiration from these great websites that feature nail art.

NAIL IT!
(nailitmag.com)

NAILPRO
(nailpro.com)

NAILS MAGAZINE
(nailsmag.com/style/nail-art)

PINTEREST
(pinterest.com/all/hair_beauty/)

BLOGS Stay up-to-date on everything that's new in the world of nail art with these bloggers.

ADVENTURES IN ACETONE
(adventuresinacetone.com)
Nail art and easy step-by-step tutorials

CHALKBOARD NAILS (chalkboardnails.com)
Innovative nail art

CHICKETTES (chickettes.com)
Gel polishes and nail art

COSMETIC SANCTUARY (cosmeticsanctuary.com)
Nail polish reviews

POINTLESS CAFÉ (pointlesscafe.com)
Nail polish reviews and nail art

SMASHLEY SPARKLES (smashleysparkles.com)
The authority on water marbling

THE DIGIT-AL DOZEN (thedigitaldozen.com)
Collaborative blog written by multiple nail artists

THE LACQUEROLOGIST (lacquerologist.com)
Nail art by Emily Draher

WONDROUSLY POLISHED (wondrouslypolished.com)
Detailed nail art

RETAILERS Purchase nail polish and nail art supplies at these online retailers.

AMAZON
(amazon.com)

ETSY
(etsy.com)

SALLY BEAUTY SUPPLY
(sallybeauty.com)

BORN PRETTY STORE
(bornprettystore.com)

HEAD2TOE BEAUTY
(head2toebeauty.com)

SEPHORA
(sephora.com)

EBAY
(ebay.com)

MASH NAILS
(mashnails.com)

ULTA
(ulta.com)

RECOMMENDED PRODUCTS

Achieve the results you want with some of the best nail care brands. Whether you shop at the drugstore, beauty specialty store, or online, there are countless brands to discover and try.

CND (available at specialty retailers and online)
Professional quality manicure and pedicure products and tools. Try their cuticle removers and natural nail files.

GLISTEN & GLOW (available at glistenandglow.com)
Online polish and nail care boutique. Try their exclusive Glisten & Glow HK Girl Top Coat, a 2-free top coat perfect for long-lasting nail art manicures, and Glisten & Glow Nail + Cuticle Balm, a jojoba oil and shea butter nail balm, perfect for maintaining healthy, beautiful nails.

KBSHIMMER (available at kbshimmer.com)
Unique handmade nail lacquer and nail care products. Independent nail polish companies are on the rise, producing innovative polish finishes and glitter mixes that you can't find in stores.

OPI NAIL POLISH (available at salons and online)
Iconic, salon-quality nail lacquer.

OUT THE DOOR (available at specialty retailers)
3-free, quick-dry top coat.

PRITI NYC (available at pritinyc.com)
Toxin-free boutique nail lacquer and treatments. Try their soy nail polish remover wipes and formaldehyde-free Strong Nail Strengthener.

WET N WILD (available at drugstores and mass retailers)
Affordable, cruelty-free nail lacquer.

ZOYA NAIL POLISH (available at zoya.com)
Toxin-free nail lacquer.

INDEX

Numbers

G

H

M

N-O

P-Q

R

S

DIY Beautiful!

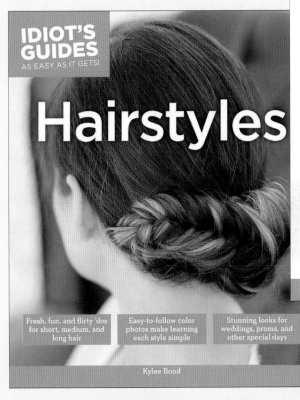

Hairstyles

IDIOT'S GUIDES
AS EASY AS IT GETS!

Fresh, fun, and flirty 'dos for short, medium, and long hair

Easy-to-follow color photos make learning each style simple

Stunning looks for weddings, proms, and other special days

Kylee Bond

9781615647040

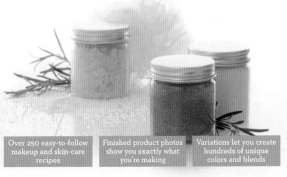

IDIOT'S GUIDES
AS EASY AS IT GETS!

Making Natural Beauty Products

Over 250 easy-to-follow makeup and skin-care recipes

Finished product photos show you exactly what you're making

Variations let you create hundreds of unique colors and blends

Sally Trew

9781615644124

idiotsguides.com

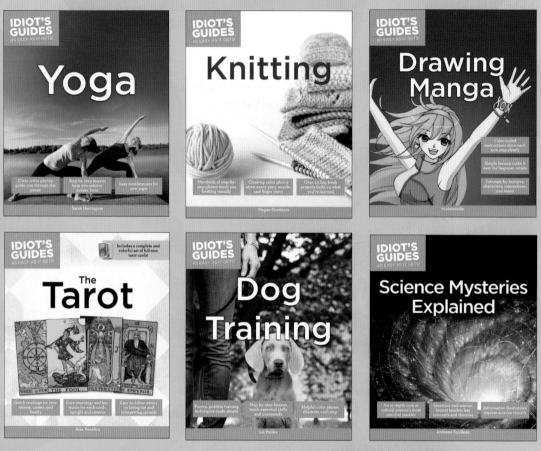
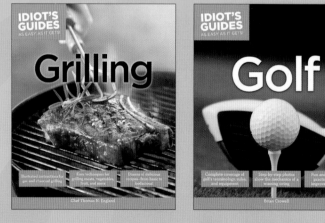